Bodies in Protest

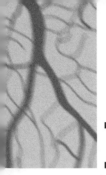

Bodies in Protest

Environmental Illness and the Struggle over Medical Knowledge

Steve Kroll-Smith and
H. Hugh Floyd

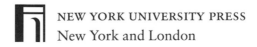

NEW YORK UNIVERSITY PRESS
New York and London

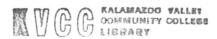
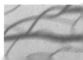

NEW YORK UNIVERSITY PRESS
New York and London

Library of Congress Cataloging-in-Publication Data
Kroll-Smith, Steve, 1947–
Bodies in protest : environmental illness and the struggle
over medical knowledge / Steve Kroll-Smith and
H. Hugh Floyd.
p.   cm.
Includes index.
ISBN 0-8147-4662-4 (acid-free paper)
1. Environmentally-induced diseases. 2. Allergy.
I. Floyd, H. Hugh, 1943– . II. Title.
RB152.K76   1997
616.9'8—dc21   97-4665
                CIP

New York University Press books are printed on acid-free paper,
and their binding materials are chosen for strength and durability.

Manufactured in the United States of America
10 9 8 7 6 5 4 3 2 1

Contents

Steve Kroll-Smith dedicates this book to his parents, Jack and Betty Smith, who in staying the course are showing their children and grandchildren the way.

Acknowledgments

A book is never written alone. Like a child, it takes a community to bring it to maturity. A research initiation grant from the University of New Orleans supported the first author through several months of interviewing. Vern Baxter, Valerie Gunter, and Susan Mann, colleagues in the sociology department at the University of New Orleans, read and commented on earlier drafts. Friend and colleague Pam Jenkins remained a patient listener to "tales from the field." Mike Grimes, a sociologist from Louisiana State University, provided insightful comments on chapters 1 and 2. Martha Ward, research professor of anthropology at the University of New Orleans, read chapters 1 through 3, attending to their symbolic, somatic arguments. Susan Kroll-Smith read each chapter from the standpoint of one versed in psychodynamics and interested in bodies and environments. Steve Couch and Phil Brown, good friends and colleagues, provided emotional and intellectual support throughout.

Several graduate students at the University of New Orleans assisted at various stages of the project. Melanie Diffendall assisted in compiling interview lists and organizing demographic data on respondents. Jennifer Boles worked on referencing and coding interviews. Molly Biehl coded interviews and prepared them for inclusion in the text. Finally, Sandra McMillan assisted in the preparation of a final draft. Jennifer Platt and Amanda Stallings from Samford University also contributed their skills to the project.

Finally, this book would not be possible without the expert help of the environmentally ill themselves. To Diane Hamilton the first author owes a particular thanks for inviting him to meetings at her house in

Baton Rouge, Louisiana. It was in the Human Ecology Action League (HEAL) group meetings that the initial, firsthand revelations of the trials, tribulations, and triumphs of living with an environmentally ill body became evident. In several interviews with Diane herself, a woman was revealed who was made stronger by a chronic, disabling illness. To the over 140 people who disclosed themselves in thoughtful narratives about their bodies, personal sufferings, and hopes for the future, we owe our biggest debt. We are privileged to have heard your stories. We hope that you find yourself and your body represented in this book. Thank you.

Preface

Another pandemic illness is emerging in American society. It is called, among other things, multiple chemical sensitivity (MCS), environmental illness (EI), and somewhat ominously, twentieth-century disease. It invites comparison with that most deadly modern pandemic, AIDS. In two important respects the terms *multiple chemical sensitivity* and *acquired immunodeficiency syndrome* are alike. In a strict sense, neither term denotes a disease at all. They both refer to medical conditions that are expressed in a complex array of symptoms and disorders. One person with MCS, for example, may experience memory loss and fatigue, while another breaks out in skin wheals and loses motor control. An AIDS patient, on the other hand, is vulnerable to a number of cancers or may succumb to pneumonia.

A second feature shared by MCS and AIDS is their common origin in environments, albeit quite different ones. It appears that HIV, the human immunodeficiency virus that causes AIDS, was confined to African rain forests until liberated by commercial deforestation practices. Indeed, Ebola, Marburg, and AIDS are, by all accounts, tropical viruses that would likely live in rain forests at no risk to humans if the forests were left uncultivated. Likewise, MCS is apparently caused by human intervention into environments. But, unlike AIDS, it is not an infectious agent freed from ancient ecosystems to hunt for human hosts. Instead, the commodities of late capitalist society, built environments, and consumer goods have unleashed this new pandemic. MCS is not a virus in search of a remedy; it is, to risk the charge of hyperbole, a somatic indictment of modernity.

While an antidote for the AIDS virus continues to elude biomedical science, it is expected that one (or more) will be discovered. The shared expectation that a drug will be found to kill the virus originates in the consensus of the medical community and the wider society that AIDS is a pathophysiological problem that falls within the boundaries of normal medicine. While the disease is an uncontested modern catastrophe, a solution to AIDS will be found without radically modifying the biomedical model. Since AIDS is successfully captured within the biomedical system, it is not likely to upset essential political and industrial arrangements. The disease, after all, is transmitted via bodily fluids and befalls individuals who make poor choices or are victims of the poor or negligent choices made by others. The tortured body of AIDS is among our modern nightmares, but it is not a new body; we understand it, even if we cannot at present cure it.

The bodies of the multiply chemically sensitive, in contrast, are medical anomalies. While the biomedical community quickly apprehended AIDS, defining it in manageable terms, MCS is demanding that the biomedical model itself change to accommodate its peculiar etiology and pathophysiology. People with MCS, for example, believe that their illness has little to do with contaminating bodily fluids but is caused, rather, by seemingly benign consumer products and supposedly safe places such as houses, car interiors, and offices. Barely discernible amounts of chemical irritants found almost anywhere in modern society can permanently change their bodies, rendering them physically unstable and emotionally exhausted. An antidote for MCS, therefore, is not likely to be found through pharmaceutical research or invasive surgeries; nothing less than changing conventional understandings of what are safe and dangerous places and things found in them will abate this illness.

Moreover, MCS is a relational illness in a way that AIDS is not. The term *relational illness* simply means the degree to which debilitating symptoms are believed to be caused in part by the personal habits and routines of people who live or work in the social circles occupied by sick people. While caring for an AIDS patient may require people to change their customs and habits, those customs and habits are not considered the causes or triggers of immunodeficiency symptoms. People with MCS, on the other hand, believe that at any moment their relative state of illness or wellness is a function, in part, of the activities and practices of others. Important, perhaps critical, to a person's management of MCS is her ability to persuade other people that they are partly responsible for her misery and must change if she is to successfully manage her symptoms. People with MCS must narrate their illness stories in order to survive.

Listen to the etiology stories and related narratives of the environmentally ill, and you will hear a new talk about a new body and its relationships to local environments. Observe their efforts to manage symptoms and pay attention to how they would rearrange the social and physical world to accommodate their disability, and you will witness the transformation of discourse into rhetoric. Ask questions about the significance of nonphysicians constructing medical explanations for their physical symptoms and miseries, and a broader, more inclusive trend in contemporary society may be discerned, one in which ordinary people are borrowing expert rhetorics, locating them in nonexpert systems, and working to politicize what is routinely considered natural.

Ironically, while AIDS will, at least in the near future, continue to devastate our lives, killing our lovers, spouses, friends, and acquaintances and mocking our weak and ineffectual attempts to control it, this most devastating of pandemics is not likely to result in profound political and industrial change. MCS, on the other hand, will claim few (if any) lives, but it will lay claim to an alternative strategy for the construction of rational knowledge in late modern society.

Introduction

In the early nineteenth century, the air of European cities was thought to be the source of infection and disease. The word *miasma* entered popular conversation and meant, quite literally, dangerous, deathlike air. It was not acute toxicity that disabled the person, but noxious exhalations from open sewers and industrial effluents that together worked in a slower, more villainous fashion. Urban air was characterized as particularly sinister, and people prone to illness were advised to spend as much time in the country as their resources would permit (Sontag 1989).

In 1880 the American neurologist George M. Beard identified a pattern of symptoms he called "neurasthenia" or "American nervousness." The reported symptoms included fatigue, short-term memory loss, and sore joints and muscles, among others. The etiology of neurasthenia, Beard argued, was none other than technological progress itself, namely, steam power, the printing press, and factories (Hileman 1991, 30).

The idea that fouled air or the achievements of modernity were the sources of disease was successfully challenged, however, by Pasteur and Koch, who discovered the role of germs in the cause of many illnesses (Dubos 1959). By the twentieth century, the medical community had abandoned the miasmic theory in favor of the germ theory. The subsequent development of the biomedical paradigm shifted attention away from an exogenous theory of disease, and an etiology that located disease origins in the physical, social, and spiritual environments, and toward an endogenous theory that located disease inside the body (Dubos 1959; Young 1976; Freund and McGuire 1991).

In the late twentieth century, however, the idea of sinister air has returned in the form of a nascent physical disorder called, among other things, environmental illness, and multiple chemical sensitivity. A growing number of people claim to be "chemically reactive." They firmly believe they are suffering from a disease caused by low-level, indeed subclinical, exposures to synthetic and nonsynthetic chemicals found in putatively safe environments. Living rooms, bedrooms, offices, stores, churches, parks, and other seemingly benign and predictable habitats are increasingly identified as chemically contaminated and pathogenic. If built environments and the products typically found in them are sources of pleasure, comfort, and symbols of success for most of us, for the chemically reactive they are often perilous worlds of debilitating health risks.

Expressed in the bodies of the environmentally ill is a blurring of the recognized boundaries between safe and dangerous places. Environments, of course, might well be a source of debilitating disease, but they are commonly recognized as *extreme* places, strikingly and conspicuously dangerous: a toxic spill, a munitions explosion, or a nuclear accident, for example. The immediate task here is to remove the body from the extreme environment to a nonextreme, safe place. The troubling message of the environmentally ill, however, is that what was once thought to be safe is now dangerous. Consider the words of a thoughtful essayist who suffers from this nascent disorder:

> The contamination of our world is not alone a matter of mass spraying. Indeed, for most of us this is of less importance than the innumerable small-scale exposures to which we are subjected day by day, year by year. Like the constant dripping of water that . . . wears away the hardest stone, this birth-to-death contact with dangerous chemicals may in the end prove disastrous. Each of these . . . exposures, no matter how slight, contributes to the buildup of chemicals in our bodies and so to cumulative poisoning. (Lawson 1993, 30)

Thus the chemically reactive propose that disease is caused by more than nuclear accidents, toxic waste dumps, deadly mold spores, or DDT. For them, a seemingly endless array of environments and common consumer items are considered serious health risks. The stocked shelves of grocery stores, drugstores, and hardware stores pose immediate health risks. Churches and synagogues harbor caustic agents that threaten to overwhelm the body. Schools might be toxic. Hospitals are potential danger zones, brimming with hazardous effluents. Even birthday presents might be brightly wrapped threats. It is as if modern material culture lies in wait to ambush the body of the environmentally ill. Writing almost two hundred years ago, Jean-Baptiste Lamarck anticipated MCS when he observed: "We die when we ingest too much of the environment" (quoted in Crumpler 1990, 13).

Multiple chemical sensitivity is the latest evolution in a series of environmental warnings and technological accidents to occur in the latter decades of the twentieth century. In *Silent Spring* (1962) Rachel Carson wrote ominously of the perils of DDT and its effects on the biosphere. In the 1970s, labor demanded that management clean up the workplace and fairly compensate the victims of factory and shop floor injuries. The discovery of dangerous chemicals under a residential community in Niagara Falls, New York, in the late 1970s changed forever the public's perception of parks, schools, and neighborhoods as environmentally safe. Love Canal alerted the nation to environmental dangers that were no longer limited to nature or industrial workplaces; now they could be found in backyards, basements, and playgrounds.

The nuclear accident at Three Mile Island, Pennsylvania, in 1979 highlighted the risks of splitting atoms to boil water. Massive cooling towers shaped, unsettlingly, like mushroom clouds, became icons of fear and distrust. The untold casualties from the Chernobyl nuclear fire in the Ukrainian republic of the former Soviet Union in 1986 confirmed the doubts and suspicions of many regarding nuclear energy. In 1976 twenty-nine people died of exposure to contaminated mold they inhaled while staying at a grand old hotel in Philadelphia. What quickly became known as Legionnaires' disease called attention to buildings as possible carriers of disease. The provocative phrase *sick building syndrome* soon entered popular conversation and increased further the number of potentially risky environments.

In the late 1980s and early 1990s EI emerged as a contentious health issue, exacerbated the debate over what are safe and dangerous environments, and provoked a political question: Who will control the definition of the human body and its relationship to the environment in the waning years of the twentieth century? This book examines this medical, social, and cultural conflict from the first-person accounts of the chemically reactive.

People with MCS narrate stories of their misfortune. They speak to themselves, to one another, and to those of us who do not dwell in their world of impairment. From our vantage point, EI begins with the simple idea that people who organize themselves around changes in their bodies are also organizing their minds to produce accounts of their miseries. Most of these accounts sound like biomedical theories of the body and its relationship to the environment. People who claim they are environmentally ill are theorizing the origins of their distress and its effects on the body, and are arguing for appropriate treatment strategies, using the complicated language of biomedicine. In this manner EI is a strategy for understanding a body that is becoming disorganized and unpredictable by providing it with a rational story to account for its untoward changes. Perhaps in theorizing its somatic distress, the self of the environmentally ill learns to live in a body that cannot live in putatively benign and safe places. Following the good advice of Susan DiGiacomo (1992), we will accord the voices of the sick people found in the pages of this book "an analytic status" (136).

This book is a story of bodies that no longer behave in a manner modern medicine can predict and control. It recounts the extraordinary efforts of people who inhabit those bodies to narrate plausible accounts of what went wrong. It is a story of ordinary people struggling to construct biomedical accounts of etiologies, pathophysiologies, and treatment regimens to explain and manage their debilitating physical and psychological symptoms. It is, in short, the story of a struggle to wrest control of medical discourse from medical science and challenge the cultural definition of the body and its relationship to modern environments.

Our interest is in both the *processes* of classification, abstraction, and cause-and-effect reasoning undertaken by laypersons who are organizing a way of thinking about the strange changes in their bodies, and the *products* of these processes, the ideas themselves. Specifically, how do people whose bodies rebel in the presence of extremely low levels of putatively benign consumer products and environments fashion accounts of their misery? And, simply, what kind of body is embedded in their accounts? How does the environmentally ill body differ from the conventional biomedical body? How are the environmentally ill using their homespun theories to effect changes in the conventional, agreed-upon boundaries between safe and dangerous spaces? Finally, and closely related to the issue of safe and dangerous, how are important institutional others (friends, physicians, bosses, governments, and so on) responding to these accounts of bodies that no longer work properly? In short, it is not MCS as a medical reality that is the subject of this work. Our focus, rather, is on MCS as a biomedical account of imperfections in built environments and their debilitating effects on the body constructed by ordinary people who are frustrated and disappointed in the profession of medicine.

Multiple chemical sensitivity is a medical conflict that throws into stark relief the recent work of Anthony Giddens (1990), Ulrich Beck (1992, 1995), Alain Touraine (1995), and other theorists of late modernity. It is almost as if the environmentally ill are self-consciously dramatizing the crises and changes proposed in their work, although we venture to guess that neither the chemically reactive nor the theorists have heard of one another. The correspondences between abstract theory on the one hand and concrete human activities on the other is rarely so direct and unmediated.

Late modernity is a world populated by expert systems, expert knowledge, and an increasing awareness among ordinary people that the world is an unpredictable and increasingly dangerous place (Giddens 1990; Beck 1992). Biomedicine is a good example of an expert system. It is a set of interrelated statuses and practices organized around scientific and technical ways of knowing that "systematically form the objects of which they speak" (Foucault 1973, 49). Theories of pathogenesis are confirmed by complex technologies designed to construct sick bodies and minds. Prescribed treatments are routinely founded on complex relationships between pharmacology and healing. It is physicians who enjoy exclusive access to this expert knowledge, and statutory authority gives their medical statements the power to create the objects of medicine.

Physicians, of course, are not interchangeable with ordinary persons. In the ideal world of the professions, "Medical statements cannot come from anybody" (Foucault 1973, 51). Ensuring that only licensed practitioners speak a language of expertise limits the use of expert knowledge to people whose identities and careers are linked closely to the interests of powerful elites. Thus, it is not surprising that expert knowledge is likely to be directed away from social criticism and toward regulating individuals. Medicine, in particular, locates individuals in the crosshairs of classificatory schemes and definitions that focus attention on their personal difficulties and shortcomings (Foucault 1973; see also Sontag 1989).

While states can use force to ensure compliance, most expert systems survive in part on the simple willingness of nonexperts to trust in their complicated and often mysterious powers (Giddens 1990). There are strong cultural pressures for people to follow the advice of their physicians, or at least not to resist receiving advice. People who narrate stories about bodies that are increasingly intolerant of ordinary places and things are routinely advised by their physicians to reduce the stress in their lives, or to medicate daily with allergy drugs, or to seek psychological or psychiatric help. The problem with this expert advice is, simply, that it doesn't work. People remain sick or become even sicker when they follow their physicians' recommendations.

Rather than rejecting biomedicine entirely, however, these people are appropriating the symbols of biomedicine—in effect, separating the physicians from their language and shifting the site of biomedical theorizing from hospitals, clinics, and offices to kitchen tables, living rooms, and patios. The sick people encountered in these pages are not abandoning expert knowledge but they are moving away from the expert system. They perceive the need for expertise at the same moment they have lost faith in the experts and their administrative worlds.

What might happen to biomedical knowledge once it is separated from the profession of medicine and relocated in mundane, ordinary worlds? One thing seems certain: the constitutive authority of physicians to create and control the objects of medicine in the interests of the state is not likely to go unchallenged. Ordinary people exercising control over medical discourse are likely to bend and twist at least a few of its paradigmatic assumptions to fashion ways of knowing that help them explain their miseries. In theorizing their somatic distress, the environmentally ill, in particular, are locating the sources of their troubles outside of themselves, in the practices and habits of intimate and institutional others. They are claiming to know something biomedical about the body and environments that is at once an explanation of chronic somatic distress and a representation of imperfections in the body politic—at once, in other words, a theory and a social criticism.

Bodies do not talk, of course. We do. But bodies do make noises, tremble, break, change shapes, and act in unusual ways. In short, our bodies invite, if not demand, someone to speak for them.[1] As bodies become increasingly exposed to environmental dangers whose immediate and long-term health effects are endlessly debated by experts, ordinary people are frequently compelled to speak for their own bodies. Problems with bodies and environments are challenging the orthodox boundaries between medical experts and lay forms of knowledge.

More generally, we might say that lay expertise is emerging as an alternative form of rationality, one that begins and ends with concrete human, indeed physical, experiences. A common denominator of these physical experiences, however, is their high degree of uncertainty, ambiguity, or, perhaps better said, mystery. If the cry "I am hungry" demands not reflection but concrete action, the cry "I am poisoned by invisible chemicals whose presence is not detectable using standard monitoring equipment" is an occasion for reflection, deliberation, sorting out what is known from what is not known, testing, drawing conclusions, and checking them against some standard of validity (Beck 1992). Not surprisingly, the "I am poisoned . . ." mysteries must be transformed into puzzles, changing their status from things that cannot be known with certainty to things that can be figured out.

The chemically reactive are not the only people who find the rational explanations of legitimate medical authorities to be fuzzy and confusing, if not incoherent, accounts of their troubles. Multiple chemical sensitivity is an example of a broader populist revolt against the hegemony of expert medical systems in what Giddens calls "late modernity" and Beck calls the "risk society." Participants in this revolt do not reject medical knowledge; rather, they refuse to allow it to be identified solely with the interests of state-sponsored professions. Participants, in other words, are likely to criticize the medical profession while appropriating its complex theories.

A recent article on the AIDS movement in the United States describes activists who

> wrangle with scientists on issues of truth and method . . . [and] seek to reform science . . . by locating themselves on the inside. They question not just the uses of science, not just control over science, but sometimes even the very contents of science and the processes by which it is produced. . . . They seek to change the ground rules about how the game is played. (Epstein 1991, 37)

In a similar manner, citizens are claiming to know about "women's health, fetal tissue research, and recombinant DNA research" (Epstein 1991, 36). The current controversy over the etiology of the unusual symptoms and diseases experienced by veterans of the Gulf War is pitting the ordinary soldier against the health machine of the Veterans Administration (see chapter 7). Workers are learning about accident rates and types of technology to argue for a safer workplace (Nelkin and Brown 1984). And the problems of chronic fatigue syndrome and repetition strain injury are sending citizens to the libraries in search of answers physicians cannot provide (Lawson 1993; Bammer and Martin 1992). The problem of MCS joins a new class of hazards that are characterized by the absence of concrete, tangible measures of cause and effect, that are not apprehended immediately but require rumination, deliberation, cogitation—in short, the construction of abstract explanations, theories if you will.

Theorizing is a task normally assigned to scientists and intellectuals, while nonexperts are likely to improvise ways of knowing that occur well below the level of genuine theory construction (Berger and Luckmann 1966). Today, however, an increasing number of average citizens are appropriating the privileged voice of the theorist to construct coherent groups of general propositions to use as principles of explanation and persuasion. Consider Ulrich Beck's (1992) rhetorical question:

> Why shouldn't laypeople—who are no longer what they used to be, namely, just laypeople, and who ultimately have to pay for all the benefits—ask questions that are forestalled by the false a priori of scientific theory, and in that way provide a critical supplement to the model of experimental testing? (55)

Problems of health and disease are only one example of a popular struggle to wrest control of a rational knowledge system from its institutional moorings and challenge society to change based on a claim to know something "true" or "scientific" about how the world works. Public hearing testimonies offered by citizens organized to define and control disposition of nuclear materials at the seventeen Department of Energy sites in the United States argue in the languages of nuclear engineering and toxicology for their version of appropriate cleanup criteria (U.S. Department of Energy 1991). Other citizens are mastering the intricacies of zoning and planning regulations to hold industrial developers accountable for various land-use initiatives involving hazardous or toxic materials (Couch and Kroll-Smith 1994; Minor 1994).

Human agency in liberal democracies has always depended on the ability of people to articulate their concerns and grievances using the discourses of civil rights. Today, however, what is just and unjust is often confounded with claims to know the world through categorization, calculation, and measurement. Civil rights, in other words, are increasingly dependent on the capacity of ordinary people to appropriate the languages of instrumental rationality and cast their arguments for equality and justice in the measured cadence of expertise.

Note, however, the distinction drawn here between acquiring expert knowledge and soliciting the counsel of experts. As people are becoming aware of their increasing dependence on expert knowledge they are also increasingly distrustful of experts. Perhaps this explains, in part, Beck's observation that "monopolies on knowledge...are... moving away from their prescribed places" and found increasingly in popular arenas (1992, 154). In this new history, to modify Bauman, "one [must] steal the expertise and play with it, boldly, one's self" (1993, 17).

In a provocative image of the problem, Ulrich Beck (1992) argues that society is changing from one in which "being determines consciousness" to one in which "consciousness determines being" (53). In the new society, class becomes less important in shaping thought and experience, increasingly displaced by the production of knowledge among confederates (arguably representing many classes) who define themselves as imperiled by unanticipated changes in the biosphere and unable to trust the opinions of experts. If consciousness, and not material circumstances, is shaping late-modern lives, it should also be recognized that somatic states and conditions are shaping consciousness, a point we will return to throughout this book.

Looking Ahead

Chapter 1 describes the conflict between the medical profession and the environmentally ill, paying particular attention to the difficulties physicians and medical researchers experience when they attempt to define MCS. While the medical profession is skeptical and uncertain regarding the idea that bodies are changing in relationship to ordinary environments, for the environmentally ill, MCS is a practical epistemology—a strategy for knowing the world that works to reduce or make manageable a human trouble. Chapter 2 examines two essential ways of talking (technical and emotive) and how they are used by the environmentally ill to transform themselves from objects of biomedicine into active agents who are inventing and constructing bodies by the skillful use of an expert language. The image of science joined with biography is an uncommon one in our society and is important to our account of MCS as a practical epistemology. Finally, we introduce three descriptive processes that account for how people become disenchanted with experts, borrow expert languages, and seek public recognition of their troubles.

Chapters 3 through 5 use narratives of the environmentally ill to describe in vivid detail the problems of living with a contested disease that challenges not only the biomedical definition of the body but commonsense thinking about the relationship of bodies to environments. In these chapters we encounter the work people do to make their obscure bodies intelligible by locating them in theories of etiology and pathophysiology that lead often to effective treatment strategies. Following Geertz's pragmatic idea, we refer to these local theories as *practical epistemologies* (1983, 151).

Chapters 6 and 7 shift attention from a phenomenological account of MCS to a consideration of its political and economic effects. Introducing the idea of representation, we look closely at those arenas of social and cultural life that are changing to accommodate and, in turn, recognize the chemically reactive body. To the extent institutional others are modifying routines or policies, passing legislation, or creating commodities to assist the environmentally ill body, MCS is becoming a disease in spite of the medical profession's current refusal to acknowledge it. In the final chapter we suggest that the amount of interpretive space created by problems with bodies and environments is growing. By *interpretive space* we mean simply the room available for theorizing. When citizens or laypersons step into this space, they appropriate the languages of expertise and join them to subjective, personal experiences to create an alternative rationality, at once a local and an abstract knowledge. A discussion of popular epidemiology suggests it is not only the individual body and environments that are opening up space for interpretation. Populations of bodies in the form of neighborhoods, communities, and so on are collectively proposing citizen theories of disease clusters and contamination.

Multiple chemical sensitivity and popular epidemiology are among a number of citizen science movements that are hinting at the emergence of a new history—not one they are making by themselves but one whose making they both illustrate and contribute to. This new history is neither modern nor postmodern. Modernity rested on a simple two-step formula: surrender the sovereignty of the personal, local, and subjective, and embrace the promises of abstract, rational knowledge administered by experts. Modernity offered little space for first-person stories. While they can entertain and are of some importance to social relationships or the occasional news stories—indeed, they are called "human-interest stories" in newspaper jargon—they could not be the basis for administrative decisions, legislation, or policy making. Postmodernity, it would seem, emerged to counter the formula for modernity by creating a privileged space for the personal narrative. In this society, self-stories displace expertise, which is shown to be just another self-story anyway, wrapped up in fancy language.

The environmentally ill and their counterparts in other citizen medicine movements are neither modern nor postmodern. They do not surrender their self-stories to the administration of medical expertise, as good moderns do; nor do they abandon this expertise to revel in the pure subjectivity of their stories, as good postmoderns do. Rather, they join the self-story to expertise, constructing narratives of their sick bodies using the complicated languages of biomedicine. In this fashion, MCS is a critique of both modernity and postmodernity and an invitation to revisit these important ideas as we think about the history we are making.

We wrote this book, in part, to make the environmentally ill more comprehensible than they now are—to make the "other," we might say, familiar. We invite the reader to enter their world, stay a while, and recognize the possibility that our species survives in part by its irrepressible drive to understand the significance of things, though agreement on what is or what is not significant often eludes us.

Part One

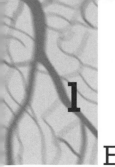

1

Environmental Illness as a Practical Epistemology and a Source of Professional Confusion

"Listen to the patient, he will tell you the source of his disease. Listen more closely and he will likely tell you how to cure him." I heard something like that once in medical school.

(The first author's family physician)

THE CONFUSING NATURE of MCS is reflected in the number of terms enlisted to describe it: environmental illness, chemical sensitivity, cerebral allergy, chemically induced immune dysregulation, total allergy syndrome, universal reactor syndrome, ecologic illness, chemical hypersensitivity syndrome, universal allergy, and, more alarming, chemical AIDS and twentieth-century disease. To simplify discussion we will use the terms *multiple chemical sensitivity,* or MCS, and *environmental illness,* or EI, to refer to the disease and the terms *chemically reactive* and *environmentally ill* to refer to the people living with the disease.

While the terms describing this medical condition vary, they converge on a number of common premises that together describe a nascent theory of the body and its relationships to the materials of modern life: office buildings, houses, shopping malls, yards and gardens, common consumer products, and so on. Importantly, what medical science knows about the etiology, pathophysiology, and treatment of EI is derived from the stories the environmentally ill tell about their bodies. Stories are all we have at the moment because there are no agreed-upon criteria for defining EI as an official medical condition and, consequently, there is no consensus regarding appropriate diagnostic protocols or treatment regimens (Ashford and Miller 1991; Bascom 1989). On the second page of their recent collaborative report, the U.S. Department of Health and the Agency for Toxic Substances and Disease Registry (ATSDR) reported that the natural history of EI describes "diverse pathogenic mechanisms . . . but experimental models for testing them have not been established (Mitchell 1995, 2).

Thus, medical researchers and physicians who accept the possibility that MCS may be a legitimate physical disorder must listen closely to their patients' efforts to explain what is wrong with their bodies. Attending to the stories of people in pain recalls the typical eighteenth-century dialogue between patient and doctor, which typically began with the question "*What* is wrong with you?" Today, however, as most of us know, a physician is more likely to ask "*Where* does it hurt?" reflecting her greater faith in sophisticated technology than in the commonsense reasoning of her patients (Foucault 1973, xviii).

But the symbols of medical technology are silent on the issue of EI. It is, rather, the phenomenology of MCS, the experiences and accounts of those living with the malady that are the primary source of knowledge about this nascent physical disorder.[1] A remarkable feature of the accounts collected for this book are their similarities, in spite of the fact that with a few exceptions the people interviewed do not know one another. Interviews with plumbers, accountants, pharmacists, postal workers, homemakers, marine captains, insurance salespeople, sugarcane workers, college professors, and others from all fifty states, with little more in common than that they all happen to be alive at the same time, consistently reveal common patterns. Discrete people, without recruitment ideologies typical of social movements, are thinking about their troubles in an essentially similar manner.

One explanation for this uncoordinated convergence in the style and product of thinking about illness is the possibility that common changes in people's bodies are shaping common thought processes. Other, arguably less sympathetic, accounts of this unorganized collective pattern are found in several academic discussions of the MCS phenomenon, including arguments that it is a form of hysterical contagion (Brodsky 1984) or chemophobia (Brown and Lees-Haley 1992). Complementing these psychosocial constructions is the unsettling idea that MCS is a pandemic outbreak of one of a number of faulty thinking disorders, including conditioned responses, symptom amplification, or displacement/avoidance activities (Simon 1995, 45; Simon, Katon, and Sparks 1990; Terr 1987).

The environmentally ill talk about a polysymptomatic disorder that starts with an acute or chronic exposure to chemical agents. Many of these agents are found in ordinary household and work environments in amounts well below recognized thresholds for toxicity. Following the initial sensitization experience(s) to a single chemical irritant, the body begins to express intolerance to an increasing array of unrelated irritants. A person with EI, for example, can react to volatile organic compounds emitted from gas stoves, dry-cleaned clothing, ammonia found in paper products, boron in cosmetics, phenol in air fresheners, and ethyl chloride in plastics, at doses that are magnitudes below those known to be dangerous. Ann became ill when she was exposed to formaldehyde in the new carpet in her office. A few days after the onset of her initial symptoms, she noticed that her body reacted aversely to her husband's colognes, her housekeeper's cleaning solvents, the painted wooden baskets hanging in her den, her laundry soap, and so on.[2]

The body's increasing intolerance to ordinary, putatively benign places and mundane consumer products is a key feature of this illness and one that baffles most physicians. "We don't dismiss these people, they are truly ill," admits a prominent allergist and medical researcher who speaks for the majority of practicing physicians, "but batteries of chemical tests can't pinpoint any specific sensitivity. Some are definitely allergic and we all agree that they are suffering, but we simply don't understand the cause of the disease as determined by medical diagnosis" (Selner 1991, 2–3). Another sympathetic but discouraging assessment concludes that "there is no laboratory test that can diagnose MCS, no fixed constellation of signs and symptoms, and no single pathogen to isolate and transmit through a cell line. . . . Even worse, some chemicals are neurotoxic and may produce symptoms that resemble anxiety attacks or mood disorders" (Needleman 1991, 33). Still more pessimistic is a public health physician who concludes that at present what is known about MCS "is insufficient to recommend programs for preventive strategies" (Bascom 1989, 36).

Adding to an already complicated theory is a premise that bodies are vulnerable to extremely low levels of chemical exposures: "below exposure levels for various chemicals established by the government, and usually below exposure levels tolerated by most people" (Pullman and Szymanski 1993, 17). This a difficult premise to test, however. If exposure levels are orders of magnitude below those deemed medically permissible, measuring concentrations of chemicals in soil, air, or water is unlikely to yield any useful information. If the concentrations are lower than permissible levels, the question still remains, How are they adversely affecting these bodies? The question is currently unanswerable empirically, though MCS suggests a theoretical rationale: Is it not possible that some bodies are more sensitive than others? Is it reasonable to sort bodies into nonsensitive, sensitive, and "hypersensitive," where sensitive bodies are more reactive than nonsensitive bodies, and hypersensitive bodies "are more sensitive than sensitive"? (Bascom 1989, 10; Ashford and Miller 1991). At least one person with EI now sorts his world into new categories: "I use to think in terms of people who are good on the one hand and bad people. Now I'm more likely to wonder whether this person is supersensitive like me or able to tolerate everything."

Complicating an already complex theory, another premise of MCS is that each chemical irritant may trigger a different constellation of symptoms in each person and that every system in the body can be adversely affected. Thus, combinations of body systems and symptoms interact geometrically, creating, at least theoretically, a seemingly endless configuration of somatic miseries (Pullman and Szymanski 1993, 17; Ashford and Miller 1991; Cullen 1987). Consider, for example, an abbreviated list of EI symptoms distributed by the Chemical Injury Information Network, an MCS support group. Among the sixty-two symptoms listed are sneezing, loss of smell, nosebleeds, dysphagia (difficulty in swallowing), dry or burning throat, tinnitus (ringing in the ears), hearing loss, hyperacusis (sound sensitivity), coughing, shortness of breath, hyperventilation, high and low blood pressure, hives, constipation, thirst, spontaneous bruising, swelling of heart or lungs, night sweats, insomnia, poor concentration, and depression (Duehring and Wilson 1994).

Robert loses his balance and becomes disoriented when he is around fresh paint, while Diane is likely to become nauseated and tired. Both manifest different symptoms when exposed to different chemical agents, challenging the biomedical assumption that each disease is caused by a specific aversive agent affecting an identifiable body system (Freund and McGuire 1991). Symptoms simultaneously involving multiple body systems, but affecting each differently, violate a foundational assumption of biomedicine that diseases are classed as specific pathological configurations (Kroll-Smith and Ladd 1993). A physician-researcher who frequently testifies against plaintiffs who claim to be environmentally ill and sue their employers for negligence in the management of a chemical work environment writes, "The persistence of symptoms, worsening of symptoms, and appearance of additional new symptoms during therapy attest to a pattern of fear of the everyday environment engendered by an unfounded perception of an environmentally damaged immune system" (Terr 1987, 693). A theory of chemically damaged immune systems, however, is only one of several pathophysiology theories of MCS, as we will see in chapter 5.

Finally, people with MCS are likely to ascribe to a treatment regimen that emphasizes avoidance and lifestyle changes rather than drugs, surgery, or other invasive therapies (Bascom 1989; Ashford and

Miller 1991; Kroll-Smith and Ladd 1993). Healing the body is specifically not an invasive procedure. Rather, healing begins with removing the offending substances from the body and working to keep those substances at a safe distance. Avoidance and self-discipline are key elements of successful coping. Avoidance measures can be as subtle as moving away from a person wearing hair spray or cologne to moving into an environment built specifically to reduce chemical exposure. Wimberly, a small town in central Texas, has gradually become a chemically free refuge for people with extreme MCS. While only a small number of the chemically reactive move to such special environments, most are forced into some form of social and spatial exile to successfully manage their symptoms.

Avoidance can also be more proactive. Increasingly, people who theorize their bodies' relationship to environments using some variant of MCS try to persuade others to change their personal habits, approach employers with specific requests that would reduce their exposure to offending substances, and appeal to local, state, and national legislatures to create "safe zones" free of dangerous chemicals.[3]

A strategy of avoidance based on escape and one based on changing habits, ordinances, or the materials of production are effectively redrawing the boundaries between safe and dangerous places, though with varying social and political effects. Families who leave Los Angeles and move high into the Sierra Madres to escape a chemically saturated world are building alternative, "ecologically safe" communities; they are not, however, directly challenging society to change. A wife who refrains from wearing a "toxic scent," an employer who moves an offending copying machine from a nearby office, and a county board of supervisors that passes an ordinance establishing a "fragrance-free zone" in the local courthouse are examples of social and legal accommodations to the environmentally ill who petition others to change. When others change, the environmentally ill stand a chance of living within society rather than merely surviving by escaping from it.

Whether they manage their symptoms by escaping society or challenging it, or some combination of the two, the environmentally ill are forced to carve up the meaning of space in a manner unfamiliar to most people. Thus, while their behavior can appear strange and untoward, perhaps insulting, to others, for them it is a reasonable response to the management of their symptoms.

~

The exact number of people who claim to be environmentally ill is not known. The U.S. Department of Health and Human Services admits it cannot estimate their numbers (Samet and Davis 1995). Commonsense comparisons, speculation, and anecdotes are the fallback strategies for calculating the scope of the problem. The Labor Institute of New York notes: "While it is clear that a significant portion of the population is sensitive to irritants such as cigarette smoke, the percentage of individuals who are significantly affected by multiple chemical sensitivities appears to be much smaller" (Pullman and Szymanski 1993, 18).

Though it does not use the term multiple chemical sensitivity, environmental illness, or any of the other variants, the National Academy of Sciences (1987) suggests that between 15 and 20 percent of the U.S. population is allergic to chemicals commonly found in the environment, placing them at increased risk of contracting a debilitating illness. The National Research Council's Board on Environmental Studies and Toxicology (1992) reports that "patients have been identified with a condition of multiple and often diverse symptoms that have been attributed to chemical agents in the environment" (5), though it does not specify how many.

Complementing this anecdotal approach to determining the breadth of the problem are several additional facts and figures that suggest that EI is more than a minor medical annoyance. A nonrandom survey of people who identified themselves as having MCS found sixty-eight hundred respondents (quoted in Ashford and Miller 1991, 5). The Chemical Injury Information Network lists multiple support groups for people with EI in forty-four of the fifty states. Support groups also meet in Finland, Germany, Australia, Canada, Denmark, New Zealand, France, Mexico, Belgium, and the Bahamas. We identified twenty-nine newsletters circulating in the United States devoted to chemicals, bodies, and the environment.

The range of demographic groups reporting the symptoms of MCS suggest it is a pandemic problem:

> A review of the literature on exposure to low levels of chemicals reveals
> four groups or clusters of people with heightened reactivity: industrial
> workers, occupants of "tight buildings," . . . residents of communities
> with contaminated soil, water, and air, and individuals who have had...
> unique exposures to various chemicals. (Ashford and Miller 1991, 3)

This list implies that everyone is susceptible to the ravages of MCS. There is some evidence to support this unsettling idea.

Industry groups estimate that over a third of new and remodeled office and storage buildings harbor indoor air pollutants sufficiently toxic to increase employee absenteeism by as much as 20 percent (Molloy 1993, 3). In addition to the building materials themselves, the Occupational Safety and Health Administration counted a minimum of "575,000 chemical products . . . used in businesses throughout the U.S." (Duehring and Wilson 1994, 4; see also U.S. Department of Labor 1988). In 1989 the U.S. Environmental Protection Agency estimated that employers lose approximately sixty billion dollars a year to absenteeism caused by building-related illnesses (cited in Molloy 1993, 3). Not every victim of a "sick building" becomes environmentally ill, of course, but "bad air" at work is a common explanation for the origin of chemical reactivity among the environmentally ill.

But the workplace is not the only source of EI. Aerial pesticide spraying, incineration practices, and groundwater contamination are among the causes of MCS in neighborhoods and communities (Ashford and Miller 1991). In addition, the U.S. Environmental Protection Agency reported that one in four people in the United States live on top of, adjacent to, or near an uncontrolled hazardous waste site (1980; see also Szasz 1994).

Finally, consider a series of troubling statistics culled from several sources:

- In 1940 the annual production of synthetic organic chemicals in the United States was 2.2 billion pounds. By 1991 it had increased to over 214 billion pounds, an increase of 200 percent in fifty years (National Research Council 1991, 21).
- "The EPA's Office of Toxic Substances is called upon to review approximately 2000 new chemical products a year" (Duehring and Wilson 1994, 4).
- The EPA can ensure the safety of only six out of six hundred active pesticide ingredients under its control (Duehring and Wilson 1994, 10).
- Less than 10 percent of the seventy thousand chemicals now in commercial use have been tested for their possible adverse effects on the nervous system and "'only a handful have been evaluated thoroughly,' according to the National Research Council" (Duehring and Wilson 1994, 4).
- The EPA has identified over nine hundred volatile organic chemicals in ordinary indoor environments including offices and houses (reported in *Delicate Balance* 1992, 9).
- Finally, an EPA Executive Summary on chemicals in human tissue found measurable levels of styrene and ethyl phenol in 100 percent of adults living in the United States. The Summary also found 96 percent of adults with clinical levels of chlorobenzene, benzene, and ethyl benzene; 91 percent with toluene; and 83 percent with polychlorinated byphenols (Stanley 1986).

There is, in short, ample opportunity for individual exposure to a seemingly endless parade of chemicals whose effects on the body are simply not known.

While it is not possible to know with any certainty how many people claim to suffer from MCS, it is reasonable to assume the number is substantial and growing. At the very least, it is possible to imagine how a person might link an array of bizarre and debilitating symptoms to a disease theory based on a premise that the body is exposed to an extraordinary number of chemically saturated environments.

EI and the Profession of Medicine

People with MCS are theorizing what makes them sick, how specifically their bodies are changed (immune system, limbic system, and so on), and what can be done to decrease or manage their symptoms. When they speak of MCS, there is often a tone of certainty in their voices. While certain, they are not arrogant, however. The surety of knowing is typically accompanied by self-doubt, anger, fear of the future, and other troubling emotions. While a chemically reactive person is reasonably confident in his theory of what is wrong with his body, why, and how he can manage his symptoms, MCS is not recognized by the profession of medicine as a legitimate physical disorder.

Indeed, medical professionals are likely to admit that currently what they do *not know* about MCS is considerably more than what they *know*. A physician's report to the Maryland Department of the Environment on the problem of EI, for example, is primarily a list of things medicine does not know about this nascent disorder, herein called chemical hypersensitivity disorder, or CHS.

- There is no single universally accepted terminology for or definition of CHS.
- There is no known cause of CHS.
- There is no prognosis for individuals with CHS.
- There are no criteria or procedures for reporting sensitivity disorders as diseases.
- There are no prevalence studies of CHS.
- It is not known if the incidence or prevalence rate of CHS is increasing.
- A "risk profile" for CHS does not exist.
- Educational materials on the subject of CHS are limited, and it is not possible to determine the accuracy of the information that is available. (Bascom 1989, 2–19)

Not surprisingly, the author concludes her report by observing that not enough is known about CHS "to recommend programs for preventive strategies. . . . There is no consensus as to the cause of CHS, the appropriate medical treatment, or the appropriate policy approach" (36–37). The U.S. Department of Health and Human Services concurs: while an increasing number of people are defining themselves as environmentally ill, the definition of MCS "is elusive and its pathogenesis as a distinct entity is not confirmed" (Samet and Davis 1995, 1). An occupational medicine researcher expresses his frustration over this elusive problem: "If the question cannot be answered as to what MCS is, how can there be approval of research protocols or acceptance of investigative results? In order to appropriately address the controversies surrounding this phenomenon we must know where we're going!" (DeHart 1995, 38).

The first official recognition of MCS was probably a 1985 report by the Ad Hoc Committee on Environmental Hypersensitivity Disorders (1985) in Toronto, Canada. Two years later Dr. Mark Cullen, a medical researcher at Yale University, published a definition of MCS based on his observations of people exposed to chemical irritants at the workplace. While his definition is the most frequently cited in the biomedical literature, it clearly expresses biomedicine's uncertainty regarding this nascent disorder:

> Multiple chemical sensitivities is an acquired disorder characterized by recurrent symptoms, referable to multiple organ systems, occurring in response to demonstrable exposure to many chemically unrelated compounds at doses far below those established in the general population to cause harmful effects. No single widely accepted test of physiologic function can be shown to correlate with symptoms. (Cullen 1987, 655)

The biomedical research community is divided over the meaning of MCS and the numbers of people who have it. For some researchers, "evidence does exist to conclude that chemical sensitivity [is] a serious health and environmental problem and that public and private sector action is warranted at both the state and federal levels" (Ashford and Miller 1991, v). For others, however, a great deal more research is needed before there will even be a consensus on a definition of chemical hypersensitivity. It is premature to classify CHS [chemical hypersusceptibility] as a purely environmental problem. . . . Health related environmental standards are based on normally accepted exposure units. They do not take into account individuals who may be sensitive to chemicals at limits far below the norm, perhaps at undetectable limits given current technology. (Maryland Department of Environment, letter to Governor Donald Schaefer, in Bascom 1989)

In striking contrast to the difficulty of the biomedical research community in reaching agreement on the meaning of MCS, the clinical medical profession speaks with one voice in rejecting the legitimacy of this proposed disorder. From its perspective, MCS is a fugitive, hopefully transitory, concoction of beliefs with no rightful claim to legitimacy.

Local medical boards reportedly threaten to censure physicians who diagnose people with MCS (Hileman 1991, 27–28). National medical societies, including the American Academy of Allergy and Immunology (1989), the American College of Occupational Medicine (1990), and the American College of Physicians (1989) officially deny the reality of MCS as a physical disorder and caution physicians not to treat patients "as if" the disease existed. The executive committee of the American Academy of Allergy and Immunology could be said to speak for the other professional medical societies in its position statement on MCS:

The environment is very important in the lives of every human being [*sic*]. Environmental factors, such as chemicals and pollutants, have been demonstrated to influence health. The idea that the environment is responsible for a multitude of human health problems is most appealing. However, to present such ideas as facts, conclusions, or even likely mechanisms without adequate support, is poor medical practice. The theoretical basis for ecologic illness in the present context has not been established as factual, nor is there satisfactory evidence to support the actual existence of . . . maladaptation. (quoted in DeHart 1995, 36)

The California Medical Association reported that "scientific and clinical evidence to support the diagnosis of environmental illness is lacking" (1986, 239). The report went on to argue that evidence supporting the existence of a low-level chemical etiology to such health problems is based on hearsay and anecdote, not controlled clinical trials (243). A study published in the *New England Journal of Medicine* found the clinical testing for MCS to be seriously flawed and the typical environmentally ill patient to be unusually stressed and personally unhappy (Jewett, Fein, and Greenberg 1990). In a report prepared for the State of Maryland, a health policy analyst summarized the hostility of the medical profession toward a biomedical interpretation of EI, observing that the "controversy surrounding the chemical hypersensitivity syndrome begins with a debate as to its very legitimacy as a distinct entity" (Bascom 1989, 8).

Results from a survey of physician members of the Association of Occupational and Environmental Clinics—the one medical society most likely to be sensitive to people who claim they are suffering from MCS—are also worth considering. First, the survey found that only 9 percent of the physician population believe EI is predominantly physical in origin. Sixty-four percent, on the other hand, believe it to be a psychological disorder (Rest 1995, 61). With this bias toward a psychogenesis model of MCS, we should not be surprised to learn that occupational physicians were more likely to consult psychiatrists and psychologists when treating a patient who theorized his misfortune as MCS (63). Similarly, 64 percent of the occupational physicians reported referring people who claim to be chemically reactive to psychologists or psychiatrists. Fifteen percent did so "always," while 49 percent did so "at least half the time" (65).

A report in the *Annals of Internal Medicine* labeled people claiming to suffer from MCS a "cult" (Kahn and Letz 1989, 105).[4] Adding insult to injury, an allergist reports that he can reduce the symptoms of the disorder by "deprogramming" patients who internalize "environmental illness beliefs" (Selner 1988). A psychiatrist writes: "In the absence of objectively verified abnormalities detected in physical examination, the illness is subjective only. . . . Multiple Chemical Sensitivity constitutes a belief, not a disease" (Brodsky 1984, 742). A study of twenty-three people who identified themselves as environmentally ill found fifteen of them suffering from a mood, anxiety, or somatoform disorder (Black, Rathe, and Goldstein 1990). The authors of this study, published in the *Journal of the American Medical Association,* conclude that all people with EI "may have one or more commonly recognized psychiatric disorders that could explain some or all of their symptoms" (3166).

Finally, Gregory Simon, another psychiatrist and coauthor of a well-known article on MCS, "Allergic to Life: Psychological Factors in Environmental Illness" (Simon, Katon, and Sparks 1990), argues that MCS is simply a product of faulty reasoning. Recalling the classic anthropological question, "Can 'primitive' people distinguish fact from fancy or do they muck around in a hodgepodge of spirits, sprites, myths, and legends?" Simon and colleagues label the environmentally ill victims of, simply put, bad reasoning. Like Lévy-Bruhl's primitive, they cannot discern what is real from what is imaginary. Thus for some experts MCS is a result of behavioral sensitization. People associate a smell or taste with a physical symptom, in spite of the fact that there is no clinical relationship between the two. For others, MCS is a consequence of a tendency to react unreasonably to physical symptoms such as a sore throat or a rash. Investing too much attention in these symptoms, they search for causes and find them in the local environment. Finally, for still others MCS is a result of a faulty mode of reasoning perhaps best called "displacement confusion." Here a person avoids thinking about the "real" causes of physical distress, unhealthy lifestyles, excessive stress, and so on, and focuses instead on modern culture's overconcern with the environmental causes of disease (Simon, Katon, and Sparks 1990; see also Simon 1995, 45).

What are we to make of this confusing array of biological and psychological accounts of EI? Those in the medical research community are more sympathetic than their counterparts in clinical medicine to the idea that MCS is a legitimate medical disorder. But research on MCS is just beginning. Indeed, as we write this book, there is not even a commonly accepted case definition of the problem. Thus medical researchers are still debating the essential question: What *is* it? The clinical medical community appears to be ahead of its research colleagues, at least in knowing what MCS is *not*. It is not a legitimate physical disorder. While there is some confusion over what MCS might be—a belief, a cult, a psychiatric disorder, or a process of faulty reasoning—it is not recognized as a physical disease by the medical profession.

Thus, what happens when a person who has been closely monitoring his body, matching symptoms with environments, and organizing his local world to make some sense of his distress visits a physician trained to look beyond a patient's account and examine the body as the source of disease?

Doctors, Patients, and Paradigm Disputes

When physicians receive patients' complaints, it is their professional responsibility to translate them into a language that is created and controlled by the normal science model of medicine. Although they use the most sophisticated medical technology and are guided by the cultural authority of biomedicine to "define and evaluate their patients' condition" (Starr 1982, 16), most physicians who treat the environmentally ill fail to heal them.

Imagine the physician presented with a patient such as Howard, complaining of nasal obstruction, sinus discomfort, chest pain, flushing hives, itching eyes, loss of visual acuity, fatigue and insomnia, genital itch, and nausea. Imagine that no accepted tests of organ system function can explain the symptoms. Imagine also that the patient is nonreactive to any conventional treatment plan the physician prescribes. The complaints persist. Finally, imagine that the patient has a theory that explains the origins of the symptoms, but that such a theory does not correspond to any of the accepted etiologies within the biomedical model. It is not unreasonable to assume that patient and physician will tire of this cycle of frustration. The physician might suggest another doctor, or the patient might simply give up and go elsewhere. Whatever happens, the bioscience model of medicine has failed to provide the means for the patient to act like a patient and the doctor to act like a doctor; that is, the physician did not heal and the patient did not recover. If the enactment of biomedicine occurs at the moment its body of knowledge encounters a body, the body of the environmentally ill obscures that moment and effectively prevents the encounter.

~

Why is the profession of medicine unable to certify MCS as a legitimate physical disorder? Perhaps it isn't one. That is the simplest answer. It is more complicated and more interesting, however, to consider MCS as a theory of the body and the environment that contests both the medical profession's responsibility to define bodies and several of its paradigmatic assumptions about disease.

First, medicine works closely with the state to define and regulate bodies in the interest of cultural and capital production (Foucault 1973; Turner 1995). Capitalism in the waning years of the twentieth century is interested in bodies insofar as they are able to work and consume, and do so in a flexible manner (Martin 1990; Harvey 1989). The healthy body, in other words, is one that goes to work regularly, purchases and consumes the products of its or others' labors, and is capable of adapting quickly to changing modes of production and skill requirements. A putative somatic disorder that denotes change in the definition of the body in its relationship to common consumer products and domestic and workplace environments, therefore, is likely to be scrutinized closely before it is officially recognized as a disease. The environmentally ill body is, of course, anything but flexible.

But something more basic than an abstract political economy is at work here.

Howard's unfortunate predicament suggests that a formidable problem for attending physicians is the result of the limitations of their diagnostic technologies in certifying something called MCS. Medical technology is built to measure and test the assumptions of the biomedical model. Among the many assumptions in this model are two that are particularly relevant to MCS. From classic toxicology comes the supposition that a relatively small number of individuals are sensitive to low, but nevertheless measurable, exposures to certain toxins. From allergy comes the classic IgE-mediated responses by atopic individuals with overactive antibodies that mistake ordinary environmental stimuli (ragweed, pollen, dust, and so on) for poison. What the biomedical model does not assume, however, is a third, entirely different, type of sensitivity.

A principal characteristic of MCS is that after the initial sensitization, there is no identifiable threshold or exposure level below which there is a negligible risk of becoming sick (Davis 1986, 12). People who identify themselves as environmentally ill report that an acute or chronic exposure to chemicals sensitizes their bodies to respond adversely to extremely low, subclinical exposures to a seemingly endless array of unrelated chemical compounds. (The term *subclinical* is used here to denote the absence of a diagnostic technology capable of identifying the quantity of chemicals that purportedly change the bodies of the chemically reactive.)

Canada's Ministry of Health concludes in a report on MCS that "affected persons have varying degrees of morbidity and no single laboratory test including serum IgF is consistently altered" (Davis 1986, 35). Acknowledging this limitation, the National Research Council (1992) concludes quite simply that the "symptomatology related to multiple chemicals is a distinct feature of [EI] patients that is not classifiable by existing criteria used in conventional medical practice" (5). Multiple chemical sensitivity, in other words, is a medical anomaly; and like all scientific anomalies it is approached as an "untruth, a should-be-solvable-but-is-unsolvable problem, a germane but unwelcome result" (Mastermind 1970, 83).

But MCS is more than an awkward fact for the profession of medicine. Indeed, medical anomalies are common. At this time, for example, the etiologies of Sjögren's syndrome and idiopathic pulmonary fibrosis are simply unknown and treatments difficult to prescribe. A new strain of tuberculosis is resisting proven antidotes and spreading to dangerous levels in urban areas. And AIDS continues its deadly course, labeled but eluding cures. But most medical anomalies, including those just mentioned, are puzzles whose solutions will not change the cultural definition of the body. Multiple chemical sensitivity, on the other hand, is more a mystery than a puzzle. If a puzzle is a game to exercise the mind by encouraging a search for the solution, a mystery admits of no solution unless the rules of the game itself are changed. More than a puzzle or awkward fact, MCS would change the rules of the game by changing what is known about bodies and supposedly safe environments.

At the heart of this undecided battle are the environmentally ill, challenging the received wisdom about the body by linking their somatic disorders to rational explanations borrowed from the profession of medicine. It is not, in other words, the languages of the occult, New Age, or Eastern philosophy that are adopted by the chemically reactive to interpret their somatic misery. It is not crystal therapy, homeopathy, past-life regression, or obeisance to self-appointed gurus that serves as a resource for knowing. Rather, these individuals are apprehending their bodies using the rational, Enlightenment language of biomedicine. If Carl Sagan (1996) truly laments the modern revolt against science and the resurgence of a "demon-haunted world," he should be pleased to hear of ordinary people who are struggling to know something logical and reasonable about their bodies.

The environmentally ill are likely to apprehend their somatic misery using the technical language of biomedicine rather than some variation of New Age knowledge for at least one rather obvious reason: they experience their bodies changing in the presence of consumer items commonly regarded as safe and in ordinary environments com-

monly regarded as benign. Consider, for example, the following field
note describing an incident that occurred during an interview with a
person who claims to be environmentally ill:

> I sat roughly twenty feet from Jack. We were in his living room. Jack's
> house is set up for someone who is environmentally ill. Air-filtering
> machines are running in several rooms. Magazines, newspapers, and
> other printed materials are noticeably absent. A plastic housing covers
> the TV screen to block harmful low-level electromagnetic waves emit-
> ted from the picture tube.
>
> I am properly washed and attired. (That is, I showered without using
> soap and am wearing all cotton that has been washed dozens of times.)
>
> Shortly after starting the interview, Jack became visibly agitated, lift-
> ing himself from side to side and up and down in his chair. Red blotches
> appeared on his arms and face. He started to slur his words. He
> explained that he was reacting to something new in the house. Since I
> was the only new thing around, he started to ask me questions: Was I
> wearing a cologne? Was I wearing all cotton? Could I have washed my
> clothes using a fabric softener? And so on. With the exception of the
> cotton question, I answered "no" to each query.
>
> His symptoms were increasing in severity. He looked at my pen and
> asked if it contained a soy-based ink. I told him I bought it at a book-
> store without checking the chemical composition of the ink. He smiled
> knowingly and asked me to put the ink pen outside. Within a few min-
> utes his symptoms subsided.

The question is not whether Jack's body changed in front of me.
It did. The question, rather, is how to interpret the change. Using a
process of elimination, Jack concluded that the one foreign item in his
house responsible for his somatic distress was an ordinary ballpoint
pen. Remember, the distance between Jack and the pen was approximately twenty feet. I asked him to explain how he knew the cause of
his symptoms was the pen and how an ink pen that was twenty feet
away could affect him so seriously. He told me about the synthetic
chemicals in ink and their particular effects on him. He explained how
the air circulator in the living room was pointing at my back and fac-

ing him. Thus, it blew the offgassing ink from the point of my pen toward him.

Jack's carefully thought-out explanation of his somatic distress struck me as interesting, if debatable. Every move in his "first-this-and-then-that" style of reasoning is grounded in a testable assumption. And Jack was not surprised when his symptoms subsided after the pen was removed from the house. "What else could it have been?" he reasoned. Jack is in the habit of theorizing his illness by constructing what for him and, at least some, others are reasonable accounts of the causes of his misery. For Jack, theorizing his illness in a language of instrumental rationality allows him to explain his body to others and, importantly, allows him to live with some degree of self-respect in a very sick body.

For some people, however, Jack's story is questionable, indeed bizarre. He tells a fantastic tale about bodies and environments. Moreover, he requests that others modify and change what have always seemed benign, if not aesthetic or pleasurable, behaviors. If they do not do so, they are implicated in the exacerbation of his illness. His spouse, a friend, the teller at the corner bank, an office mate, a sociologist who requests an interview, and even a complete stranger become potential sources of acute, debilitating distress; once safe, innocuous places are now health risks. Jack approaches his new life as environmentally ill armed with an explanation of his body and its complicated relationship to common consumer items and local places.

For Jack, MCS is not only a chronic sickness; it is a vocabulary of motives, a type of "justificatory conversation" (Mills 1967). The "truth" of Jack's story can be measured in the degree of accommodation people make to his disabled body. The success of the environmentally ill in convincing others of the threat to health posed by mundane environments and ordinary consumer items, while also claiming the right to institutional recognition of their sickness, depends, as we will see, on the ability to borrow liberally from the vernacular of biomedicine to lobby for the transformation of their illness experiences into an official disease.

Environmental Illness as a Practical Epistemology

What is true for Jack is true for thousands of people living with bodies they believe are made sick by the environment. Multiple chemical sensitivity is a nascent theory of bodies and environments. It is a novel form of theorizing the relationships of people, bodies, and environments that unhinges an expert knowledge from an expert system and links it to historical and biographical experience to make a particularly persuasive claim on truth. It is a local knowledge, constructed in situ by people who believe they need to reorganize how they think about their bodies and the environments that surround them. Power may be a source of knowledge in a post-Enlightenment world, as Foucault announced, but rational knowledge nevertheless remains a powerful social resource. Indeed, if modernity has a commandment it is to *act in accord with reason.*[5] Rational knowledge is always an assertion of the correct, the logical, the appropriate. If something is accepted as true, then rational organizations and human beings are expected to organize their conduct to reflect this truth. Rational knowledge "is always a legitimating idea" (Wright 1992, 6). In fact, it is self-legitimating insofar as its claim to truth rests on the premise that "all that is real is rational, [while] all that is rational is real" (Lyotard 1992, 29). Thus, to accept someone's account as rational is to tacitly commit to the line of conduct and belief embedded in that account, or to risk the charge of behaving irrationally.

Society places a particular premium on the authority of rational knowledge to regulate nature and health (Wright 1992; Touraine 1995; Freund and McGuire 1991). Knowing nature, including the nature of the body, depends upon a detached observer trained to identify by means of calibrated instruments the intricacies of biological and physical systems. It is not surprising, therefore, that the privilege of theorizing the body and its relationship to the environment is limited to people educated and licensed by the state to speak the language of biomedicine.

It is the chemically reactive, however, and not the medical profession, who are classifying and explaining their anomalous medical condition. People who identify themselves as environmentally ill are shifting the social location of theorizing bodies and environments from medical professionals to nonprofessionals, from experts to nonexperts. When theorizing somatic distress in the language of biomedicine shifts from experts to laypersons, it enters a new social world, one governed by purposes other than institutional legitimation. Thus, when expert knowledge is separated from its institutional moorings and taken into another world, it is likely to be fashioned into a new cultural tool, or, as Geertz (1983) would have it, a "practical epistemology" (151). While Geertz leaves this term purposively vague, we will mean by it a technical, rational way of knowing that is responsive to the immediate personal and communal needs of nonexperts. A practical epistemology, in other words, joins the world of personal and biographical experiences to forms of instrumental rationality. Jack's story of an ballpoint pen is a good example of a practical epistemology at work. The state-sponsored owners of biomedical knowledge most likely would dismiss his account as nonsense, if not evidence of delusion. Jack, however, borrows liberally from biomedicine and common sense to conceptualize and organize a world of signs that allows him to explain and respond to a body his doctors cannot understand.[6]

It is not a desire to engage the medical profession in spirited debate, however, that is motivating the environmentally ill. A person who confiscates the privilege of physicians to explain bodies in relationship to environments is thinking about something more elemental than an epistemological dispute, to wit, simple survival. "We are always searching for ways of explaining to others what we have," acknowledges a woman with MCS, "and I guess . . . to explain to ourselves too." An engineer with a long history of the disorder recalls that "at first it was a search for a vocabulary that could express what I, or I guess my body, was going through. Crazy-sounding words like 'toxic toys' and 'VOC reactivity' became a standard way of talking for me; and still is." The efforts of the environmentally ill to find the words necessary to apprehend their misery constitute one part of this study; the specific ways they use these words to alter the social landscape and change their life circumstances constitute the other.

The environmentally sick use their theories of the body and environment to ask others to understand their misery, alter their behaviors, allocate time and money, and, generally, change the world to accommodate their illness. Specifically, rational theories of chemical reactivity become rhetorical idioms for assigning moral significance to previously amoral behaviors or habits and traditionally inconsequential environments and consumer products. When a chemically reactive husband requests that his wife of twenty years refrain from using her usual dry skin lotion, she will probably ask him why. If we listen to his reply, we are likely to hear a biomedical explanation of the effects of such chemicals as butylene glycol or phenoxyethanol on his immune system or his central nervous system. Whatever the particularities of his response, he is likely to make a causal link between chemicals in the lotion and his somatic troubles. In this fashion, what he knows about his illness becomes a lingual resource for both managing his somatic distress and critiquing behaviors, products, and environments that are routinely defined as appropriate, safe, and benign.

In theorizing the origins, pathophysiology, and effective management of their illness, the environmentally ill understand why their symptoms intensify and subside in accordance with the presence or absence of mundane consumer items and the personal habits and practices of people around them. Knowing what makes them sick and learning to avoid debilitating symptoms are cognitive resources for personal survival. With these resources these individuals can inhabit bodies that are routinely out of control with some degree of self-assurance.

Among its many manifestations, MCS is a dispute over the privilege to render a rational, in this case biomedical, account of a disabled body and the peculiar content of that account. It is a dispute over the ownership of expertise. It is a story about how institutions learn in a historical period wherein nonexperts wield languages of expertise to persuade influential others to modify their habits, regulations, and laws.

Narratives of the Environmentally Ill:
A Word about Methods

It is said that human misery is bearable only if we can tell a story about it. Perhaps it is because each of us is a storyteller that our lives have a measure of coherence and clarity. Life without narrative would be discontinuous, formless, seemingly random. Narrators create story lines, linking occurrences and ideas into plots, and give time and space a linear order. Moreover, "Personal experience must be assigned a central role in accounting for the understandability," and, we would argue, origin, "of theoretical categories and concepts" (Calhoun 1995, 86).

Except for those whose symptoms are truly severe, who cannot write or talk without considerable discomfort, most people with MCS are willing to talk about their distress. To learn about the experiences of the environmentally ill, the first author attended an environmental illness support group for approximately ten months and conducted separate interviews with each of the four members who regularly attended the group. Each person was interviewed on several occasions, and a biography of his or her illness experience was constructed. Illness biographies were written in this fashion for twelve additional people with MCS who were not members of this support group.

To provide a rough check on the reliability of these illness biographies, we subscribed for two years to four nationally circulated newsletters distributed by organizations for the environmentally ill: *Our Toxic Times*, the *Wary Canary*, the *New Reactor*, and *Delicate Balance*. We searched these documents for personal accounts of the origins of the illness, its pathophysiology, and suggested treatment regimens. Comparing the newsletter accounts with our illness biographies, we found striking similarities in the interpretive strategies people use for understanding their bodies and environments. Next, we examined two biographies written by people with EI (Lawson 1993; Crumpler 1990) and again found considerable overlap in the types of explanations typically used to make sense of bodies unable to live in ordinary environments.

Reasonably confident that the patterns of theorizing MCS discovered in the initial interviews and confirmed in newsletter accounts and biographies were generalizable to the population of people who are chemically reactive, we obtained the membership directory of the Chemical Injury Information Network. While no list can be representative of the universe of the environmentally ill, this directory is the most exhaustive list we found, and perhaps the most exhaustive list in existence. It identifies people with MCS in every state of the Union and eleven foreign countries.

We constructed a simple, open-ended questionnaire designed to solicit information on how people experienced the illness and what specifically they thought about it. We mailed this questionnaire to seventy-five people listed in the membership directory. We also asked several newsletters to print a short notice announcing our study and directing people who were interested in participating to write or call. Between the seventy-five questionnaires mailed to directory addresses and the appeals in the newsletters, we obtained an additional 147 interviews. The quality of these interviews varied. Some people responded in short, curt sentences to each question, making it difficult to learn much from their answers. Responses to 42 interviews were too cursory to be of much help.

Other people wrote between ten and twenty pages—essays steeped in reflection and pain. Still others answered the questionnaire in five to ten pages. Narratives of this length were brimming with insights into how people organized their thoughts to apprehend their miseries. Through this technique we obtained 105 interviews. Combined with the 16 interviews we conducted during the first several months of work, we collected a total of 121 usable interviews.

In addition to the interviews, we searched Med File and other library databases for medical studies of MCS. We also purchased the

Chemical Injury Information Network's bibliography on toxic chemicals and human health, which contains 1,106 entries. These secondary materials were also treated as stories of the illness.

Finally, we took our emerging conclusions back to several of the environmentally ill to ask for their comments. While a few people did not see the political importance of this type of work, expressing some disappointment that it was not a forthright call for public support, others found our story personally affirming, validating their hard-fought claim to know something important about modern bodies and environments. We are pleased to report that no one with EI who commented on our story disagreed with it.

While it is the stories of the environmentally ill that interest us, we are ever mindful of the importance of these stories to the identities of the narrators. And we are also mindful of the importance of these stories to the success of this project. The real strengths of this book are not found in our abstract musings (though we hope some readers find them useful) but in the compositions of the environmentally ill, their often insightful and always revealing accounts. We were privileged to hear and read these stories and report them in this book.

Chapter 2 continues our discussion of MCS, practical epistemology, and social critique. It develops further the conflict between the environmentally ill and the medical profession, and places this conflict in a broader historical movement identified by Alain Touraine as the return of the Subject (1995).

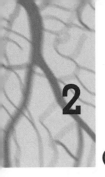

2

Chemically Reactive Bodies, Knowledge, and Society

What will become of . . . thought itself when it is subjected to the pressure of sickness?

(Nietzsche 1987, 34)

MULTIPLE CHEMICAL SENSITIVITY, at its core, is a dispute over knowing. It is a dispute over what will count as rational explanations of the relationship of the human body to local environments. One stake in this struggle is the privilege to render an authoritative explanation of the body and its relationship to the environment by, in part, accessing and applying the language of biomedicine; while the outcome may not change the traditional organization of rational knowledge, it will at the very least suggest an alternative. Also at stake in this dispute are the cultural understandings of what are safe and what are dangerous places. If social order depends in part on tacit agreement among participants that the world is divided into places to avoid and places to inhabit, MCS portends a reordering.

At this moment the dispute is little more than a skirmish of words waged between outlying detachments of opposing forces. The chemically reactive on one side, armed with their somatic experiences, borrowed biomedical interpretations, and a profound determination, look across the "no-man's-land" at the profession of biomedicine, armed with the authority of science and the state to control the definition of disease and pronounce bodies sick or well. Each side is supported by important confederates.

Siding with the chemically reactive are dozens of physicians who accept the idea of EI in spite of the resistance of their medical societies, several biomedical researchers who are working to document the physiological basis for the disorder, and an unknowable number of ordinary people who believe local environments can make people sick. Allied with the medical profession are such powerful groups as the Chemical Manufacturers Association, the Pharmaceutical Manufactures Association, and the health insurance industry.

The state's interest in promoting the use of chemicals is not hard to figure out. Approximately 80 percent of the commodities in this country are manufactured through some type of industrial chemical process (Chemical Manufacturers Association 1994). Americans bought a record high $47 billion in tobacco products in 1995 and also a record $86 billion in prescription and nonprescription drugs (*World Almanac* 1997, 150). In 1995 the U.S. Department of Commerce reported export sales of chemicals for manufacturing and chemical commercial products in excess of $50 billion. Organic and inorganic compounds alone accounted for $21 billion, while cosmetics and plastics totaled almost $19 billion (*World Almanac* 1997, 241). Also in 1995, the U.S. produced 71.16 quadrillion Btu of energy (a quadrillion is 1 with fifteen zeros behind it). Of that number, 57.40 quadrillion Btu were produced by fossil fuels (*World Almanac* 1997, 235). Finally, over a million people work in the chemical industry, including 78,400 scientists and engineers. Women make up 30 percent of the work force (*Chemical and Engineering News* 1994, 29).

Assume for the moment that society determines the knowledge claims of the environmentally ill to be true. Assume people really do become sick from exposure to a seemingly endless array of chemicals found in ordinary environments. Assume the chemicals that cause illness are present in the environment at orders of magnitude lower than current regulatory levels. Moreover, assume that exposure to one chemical compound sensitizes the body to an array of unrelated chemical compounds. Finally, assume any body system is subject to the disease. If these assumptions are true, what is at stake is more than the public right to assign a rational explanation to a human trouble. At stake in the struggle to theorize a new relationship of the body to the environment is the vast process of chemical production, disability rights legislation, housing, commercial and public building construction codes, personal habits and codes of conduct, and local, state, and federal tolerance regulations, among other significant societal changes.

Consider the account of one environmentally ill woman who struggles to reduce the number of chemical agents that trigger her symptoms:

> I stopped coloring my hair, stopped having my nails done, and stopped wearing makeup, as the petrochemicals made my eyelids swell, the tissue around my eyes dry out, and my eyelids crusty. I haven't sat on my living room chairs and couches since 1989. They are foam filled and polyester covered. I sit only on cane Breuer chairs in my own home. Shower curtains, plastic implements, plastic bags, and plastic wrap for foods are out. I avoid plastic- and polyester-covered chairs whenever possible. This, of course, is almost impossible to do in our world. . . . I gradually eliminated the restaurants and auditoriums I would normally frequent, as the chemically treated air hurt a gland in my neck. I now never go to . . . theaters, movies, concerts, or plays, or into any commercially air-cooled or heated environment. I rarely go into stores of any kind as the chemicals in the treated air cause me pain which lasts for days after, and further open me to reactions from other sources. . . . This is not an environment I can tolerate.

This account portrays a body unable to tolerate routine beauty techniques for making it attractive; a body that severely reacts to ordinary commercial furniture designed to offer it at least a modicum of rest; a body that responds violently to air passed through conventional heating and cooling systems designed to make it more comfortable; and a body that is intolerant of the seemingly countless products lining the shelves of stores and markets. It is as if this body is in protest against the products of modernity and, in its distress, is calling for a radical change in the conventional boundaries between safe and dangerous. If the built environment, in combination with any consumer item that is made with a chemical compound, renders the body chronically sick and unable to work or consume, nothing less than the transformation of material culture is warranted. Resistance to the cultural legitimation of this new and troublesome body is hardly surprising.

Moreover, if the environmentally ill body portends a social transformation in production and consumption patterns, it also threatens the delicate filigree of personal habits and tastes, and their mutual confirmation in the highly stylized world of intimate and casual relationships. In the presence of one another, we depend on a shared, unspoken sense of what may be done or said without giving offense or committing an impropriety. For the chemically reactive, however, simple expressions of good taste and regard for others may become the sources of debilitating somatic distress. A man in his early thirties remembers

> asking the people in my office to stop putting on so much cologne and perfume; I asked my office partner to stop using starch in his shirts. . . . My mom was willing to use another bathroom air thing (freshener) but my dad thought all this was much too strange. . . . I know it sounds strange but these things make me sick.

Somewhat indelicately, a more assertive woman reminds people around her, "Perfume causes brain damage. Think before you stink."

The judges who decide the winner of these skirmishes are arrayed throughout society, from intimate others, friends, work associates, and strangers who encounter the chemically reactive to municipal, county, state, and federal governments that are petitioned to accommodate them. These official and unofficial judges hear both accounts, the marginalized voices of the environmentally ill and their allies on one side and the powerful voices of medicine and trade groups on the other, supported by the suasive plea of an internalized culture that pronounces the domestic environments and products of modernity "safe" for human use. The important question is whether or not people and organizations are willing to change their behaviors regarding bodies and environments based on stories by nonprofessionals who borrow from the vernacular of biomedicine to fashion explanations of the origin of their troubles. If there is change, it is in opposition to the medical profession that refuses to acknowledge the legitimacy of environmental illness as a bio-organic disorder. If there is evidence that people and especially organizations are listening to the stories of the chemically reactive and modifying social and physical environments to assist them in coping with their troubles, then an arguably new form of social learning is surfacing, one in which organizations are bypassing a profession as a source of knowledge and modifying their practices in accord with citizens' professionally discredited accounts of bodies and environments.

This complicated conflict over knowing, embedded in the controversies surrounding MCS, begins with the body. To paraphrase Lévi-Strauss, the chemically reactive body is good to think and talk; indeed, its peculiar somatic changes insist on thinking and talking. People with MCS are forced to think about why their bodies change in the presence of common consumer products and ordinary environments; and they are often forced to explain these peculiar somatic changes to skeptical others.

Two Ways of Talking and Thinking, and the Reappearance of the Subject

We can think about our bodies because we both *are* bodies and *have* bodies (Berger and Luckmann 1966). The question, "How do we have bodies?" is routinely answered in sociology with some variant of the word *symbol*. We "have" bodies because we talk about them.

Indeed, bodies are fabricated in talk; they are, literally, figures of speech, tropes, embodied conversations, social constructions. Many conversations about the body are occurring simultaneously, however, some more privileged than others. The power of physicians and medical researchers is embedded in their use of biomedical talk to promote a culturally preferred account of the body and disqualify other accounts. To the profession of medicine society has given the right to author the body: to pronounce it legally alive, to name its systems and diseases, to control its capacity to labor by defining when it is sick and when it is well, and, finally, to pronounce it legally dead. From the birth certificate to the death certificate and everything in between, biomedicine is charged by the state with writing the somatic text.[1]

Consider, for example, a proud father who looks at his newborn daughter and observes, "She has my eyes and nose," and thus locates her body in his lineage. Important as this moment is in the life of the father and daughter, of equal or greater importance is the issuance of a state birth certificate signed by a physician that officially recognizes the infant body as living and legally belonging to the father who gave her the eyes and nose and the mother who birthed her. In the absence of state certification of the live body of the infant, the date of birth, and her legal father and mother, recognizing a similarity between her nose and that of an adult would not be sufficient to establish paternity.

Two strategies for knowing the body are evident in the configuration of the father, the infant, and the state that are important in understanding the epistemological controversy over MCS. The father apprehends the physical features of his child in talk that embeds them both in a familial world supported by history and emotion. In this fleeting moment, everyday language about the body links two subjects to a past, present, and future based on reciprocal feelings and expectations. This is truly *the* common language, a dramatic vocabulary creating and mediating attitudes, history, and community to fashion communal relationships governed by common sentiment and reciprocal expectations about behavior.

A state's bureau of vital statistics, on the other hand, issues a certificate that literally licenses the body but does so anonymously, abstractly, without face, if you will. It separates the persona from the soma and locates the body in demographic and numerical coordinates. This second talk about the body is guided by technical rules, not social norms. Its goal is the elimination of attitudes and other emotional factors that might complicate an objective location of the body in society. If the communal world is constructed through a dramatic vocabulary, the biomedical world is possible only by avoiding drama. When experts speak, scientific-technical talk works to eliminate emotion while providing, in Kenneth Burke's words, the "name and address of every event in the universe" (1973, 88).

While both talks are symbolic conversations, biomedical talk is presented as context-free, that is, ahistorical and apolitical, a "natural fact." It does not construct and sustain existential experiences; rather, it claims to mirror external reality. Diseases and treatments are discovered by the languages of anatomy, physiology, hematology, immunology, and so on. The body is a materialist product of these vocabularies, unencumbered by experiential or communal ways of knowing.

Alain Touraine would likely find our example of the father with his newborn and the bureau of vital statistics an apt illustration of his recent theory of modernity. The foundation of modernism, he contends, is the separation of the ordinary person from the instruments of rationality (1995, 219). Modernity, he argues, suffers from a cultural bipolarism, "a divorce between the world of nature, which is governed by the laws discovered and used by rational thought, and the world of the Subject" (57). Personal identity, biography, the emotive and affective culture of the individual are isolated from a managerial power legitimated by a claim to efficiency-based instrumental reason. When the world of technical rationality is dissociated from the world of subjectivity, "reason becomes an interest of might" and no longer the measure of a just and equitable society (5).

Touraine's Subject, the person who dissolves the chasm between instrumental rationality and communal, experiential history, figures prominently in the narratives of the environmentally ill. People who explain the origins of their somatic problems in chemically saturated environments are, to borrow an image from Geertz, constructing illness narratives "ostensibly scientific out of experiences broadly biographical" (1983, 10). A chemically reactive person invents and constructs a body by the skillful use of a technical language that helps him adapt to a world he no longer assumes is safe. The image of science joined with biography is an uncommon one in our society and is important to our account of environmental illness as a practical epistemology.

Recall the example of the father and the newborn in contrast with the bureau of vital statistics; while biography is created in ordinary speech that embeds both father and daughter in a common culture and history, in an entirely different and anonymous act the newborn is officially registered and classified as alive and belonging to a mother and father through a formal certification process that is nothing if it is not objective, rational, and independent of social involvements. What makes the illness narratives of the environmentally ill unique is their pattern of joining these two traditionally separated strategies for apprehending the world. Without exception, the illness stories of the chemically reactive collected for this book weave together the pain, loss, embarrassment, and challenge of a debilitating chronic illness not recognized by the profession of medicine, with a complex account of its etiology and pathophysiology, and frequent mention of sophisticated strategies for avoiding reactions and managing symptoms. Consider the following narrative.

An EI Narrative

Joan calls herself multiply chemically sensitive. Unable to use common cleaning products without experiencing debilitating headaches, nausea, and heart palpitations, she found baking soda comparatively nontoxic and buys it in bulk at her local grocery store:

On one occasion I was bringing a five-pound box of baking soda to the checkout line and my body began to react violently to something or someone in the store. I responded by pulling a cotton bandanna from my pocket and wrapped it around my nose and mouth, tying it in back of my head. I approached the checkout line. Now picture this. I am trembling, my face is masked, and I am breathing hard. Several customers looked at me and stood aside, leaving me staring, with my mouth and nose covered by a black bandanna, at the cashier.

I told the cashier that I was multiply chemically sensitive and my body was reacting to the store. I gave them my standard line: "I'm sorry for the confusion. I have environmental illness. Something happens to me when I get around certain chemical products. As you can see, my body shakes and my breathing becomes difficult. The mask blocks some of the toxins." I remember my symptoms steadily intensifying. Talking became difficult. My mouth refused to form the words I needed to speak. I was unable to grasp my wallet in my purse because my hands were trembling uncontrollably. I handed the purse to the cashier who found the wallet and rang up the sale.

I asked the cashier to call the store manager. I tried to explain to him that I drove to the store but could not drive home. At this point in my reaction, I could not hold my package or my car keys in my fingers. The manager wanted to call an ambulance. I told him that an ambulance and an emergency room would make me more sick than I was at the moment. I told him, "This is going to sound dumb, but ambulances and hospitals are full of chemicals and I know I will get sicker. I need to get home where I can take care of myself." I asked the manager to call me a cab and ask for a smoke-free cab. He took the initiative, however, and personally drove me home.

A few days following Joan's emergency at the grocery store, she wrote the store manager a thank-you card. She remembers trying to explain her problem to him so he would understand that she was "not crazy and not blaming the store." She wrote:

I have a new disease called environmental illness. I got it when I was
exposed to the chemicals 2,4-D and Diazinon while spraying my house
for fleas. The chemicals damaged my immune system and I get reactions
now to almost everything around me, but I am learning how to control
them. . . . I know I acted crazy in your store, but it is due to the chemicals. I don't mean to say your store is contaminated. I just can't tolerate things like I use to. Doctors don't believe I get sick from chemicals
like those in your store. But I do.

If the Cartesian revolution successfully silenced the authorial voice
of the body, rendering it a mechanical thing, in a passing moment in a
nondescript grocery aisle, Joan's body found a voice, its own. Giving
voice to their bodies, however, is a necessity for the environmentally
ill. As exemplified in Joan's predicament, the chemically reactive are
frequently required to tell illness stories while in acute states of distress and dependent on the help and understanding of others. It is in
this manner that illness narratives become a claim on other people by
describing new and disturbing relationships between bodies and environments.

Several observations are suggested in Joan's emergency in the grocery store and her situated explanations of her body's failure to adapt
to this mundane setting. First, it is possible to account for Joan's illness narrative as a theory about her body in relationship to the environment. She uses a coherent group of propositions regarding the
relationship between pesticide exposures and her immune system to
account for her body's inability to adapt to routine, putatively safe
environments, such as grocery stores and hospitals. Grocery stores,
and perhaps to a lesser extent hospitals, are not routinely experienced
as sources of acute illness. While someone may question the health
effects or safety of a specific item on the shelves, most people experience grocery stores as safe, domestic environments. Joan's somatic
failure, of course, may be understood as having nothing to do with the
store. Her symptoms suggest several possible standard biomedical

explanations, including grand mal seizures, epilepsy, or hysteria, that locate the causes of her distress in the body or the mind and not the immediate environment. Joan's theory, however, stresses her belief that it was the grocery store that made her sick.

Moreover, if we examine Joan's narrative, it is possible to discern a theory of disease etiology and pathophysiology. Joan theorizes that the chemicals 2,4-D and Diazinon are the source of her illness. Her exposure to these chemicals was subclinical, or below measurable levels using standard diagnostic technology. Nevertheless, her symptoms started within a few days of treating her apartment with an aerosol flea spray. The time association was important to Joan in figuring out the source of her illness. Another factor that proved important in Joan's theorizing the source of her sickness were the accounts of other people's adverse reactions to 2,4-D and Diazinon found in newspapers and newsletters and through word of mouth. Finally, Joan clung to her etiology theory with increasing tenacity as three physicians representing three different medical specialties could find nothing physically wrong with her. When the last physician she visited suggested a psychiatric evaluation, Joan ignored the suggestion and instead joined the National Coalition against Pesticides to, in her words, "become smarter than the doctors. . . . If my explanation wasn't better than theirs I was afraid people would call me crazy like the doctors thought I was."

Joan's theory of MCS also included an account of its pathophysiology and treatment regimens that worked to reduce her symptoms. Convinced the pesticides started her illness, Joan felt she also needed to know how they adversely affected her body. She talked with a nurse who lived in her neighborhood, who suggested the problem might be in her immune system. She read a *Newsweek* article on the immune system and watched a television special on AIDS. When she heard the phrase "chemical AIDS" in a National Public Radio report on EI, she concluded that the pesticides damaged her immune system and thus weakened her body's ability to fend off chemicals. Finally, while Joan is unable to find a cure for her MCS, she has developed several strategies for managing her symptoms, most of them based on avoiding those places and things that make her sick.

Is Joan's theory of MCS defensible? Perhaps not from a strict biomedical perspective. Her exposure to the pesticides was far below the threshold for acute toxicity. Assuming for the moment that she was exposed to sufficient levels of 2,4-D and Diazinon to cause an acute response, biomedicine cannot explain her subsequent sensitization to an array of unrelated chemicals. Finally, at least a few of her symptoms invited a psychosomatic interpretation.

On the other hand, Joan's account of her body is founded on the assumption that there is a natural world that can be examined. Through careful consideration of her symptoms, her experiences, and a knowledge of the (popular) literature, she has constructed a theory of her body and its adverse relationships to what were once safe and secure environments. Finally, she has tested her theory by organizing her life to avoid these environments while developing strategies for responding to stressful situations, such as the incident in the grocery store. Joan's capacity to control the definitions, meanings, and behaviors of her disability through the reflexive use of a homespun theory is a pragmatic argument for investing some faith in her ideas about her body and environments. The important question of what criteria should be used to discern the validity of MCS illness narratives is addressed in later sections of the book. At the moment it is necessary to focus on the unique features of Joan's theory about her body and environments.

Changing the Social Location, Definition, and Consequences of Expert Knowledge

Joan's theory encompasses three interrelated ideas—*social location, social definition,* and *social representation*—that work together to represent the outlines of an alternative strategy for creating and politically employing instrumental, rational knowledge in modern society. As we have defined the term here, constructing a practical epistemology may be said to begin when people appropriate a language of expertise and organize their personal lives around it. It becomes a unique way of knowing insofar as people modify and change its conventional strategies for defining and organizing. Finally, a practical epistemology becomes politically interesting when sectors of society are persuaded to change policies and habits in response to languages of expertise wielded by nonexperts who claim to know something new about the world. Consider first the idea of social location and expert knowledge.

Social Location

State-sponsored theorizing about the body and its relationship to disease and the environment is the right and obligation of the medical profession. A distinction routinely made in medical anthropology between illness and disease recognizes the unequal positions of the physician and the patient in explaining and treating sick bodies (Atkinson 1995). *Disease* is a politically powerful word controlled by the profession of medicine to classify bio-organic states of the body as unable to work properly, that is, to produce a day's labor. To have a disease is to be officially certified as unable to work at full capacity, or perhaps at all. To be designated as diseased may carry a substantial social penalty (witness the AIDS pandemic), but it is more likely to demand consideration and understanding on the part of others. Disease is, in one important sense, a rhetoric of entitlement. A state-sponsored definition of a pathogenic body pressures people and organizations to relieve a person from some (if not all) social responsibilities.[2] Without a physician's certification that the body is in a state of disease, a person who claims to be sick is likely to meet with skepticism, if not charges of malingering.

If physicians control the word *disease,* sick people are said to control the word *illness,* or the subjective awareness and meanings associated with a sick body. From the vantage point of disease, illness is a residual category. It is a necessary, but rarely privileged, concomitant of the simple fact that people *are* bodies and *have* bodies. Illness is not meant to signal a theory of etiology, pathophysiology, or treatment, for these represent the fact that people are bodies; rather, it is a cluster of words that locates sickness in meaningful social and historical arrangements, an anthropological necessity based on the fact that people have bodies and thus are required to attribute a meaning to them.

While it is true that, from the position of the state, illness is of secondary or minor importance in the classification and management of disease, it nevertheless suggests that authority over the body's problem is not in the sole possession of the physician. The ideal case, of course, is one of symmetry between the physician's assignment of a disease classification and the patient's acceptance of it; here, disease and illness merge, with one becoming, for all practical purposes, indistinguishable from the other. Perhaps the general stability of the medical profession is related, at least in part, to the observation that in this case the ideal approximates the real. A less than ideal case is a physician's diagnosis that is resisted by the person; here other institutional authorities (parents, spouses, employers) may be called upon to persuade him or her to "be reasonable and follow the doctor's recommendations."

Arguably the most disquieting case of all is the person who defines himself as sick although a physician is unable to certify that a physical basis for a disorder exists. Here a request for a disease classification is officially denied, leaving the person with a choice: to accept the authoritative account that "nothing physically unusual is happening" or to maintain a "something physically unusual" stance. The first choice may or may not be troublesome for the person, but it is unlikely to become a social issue. After all, the appearance is that the doctor and patient each performed their respective roles in a respectable fashion. If the patient later dies because of the physician's failure to diagnose in time, society is able to sanction or discredit the physician while simultaneously affirming the competence of the medical profession. The choice to adhere to the "something physically unusual" claim in spite of the doctor's opinion, however, places the person in the unenviable position of scrambling to find resources to persuade others that the medical community is wrong and he is right, and, moreover, that he should be accorded the social and moral status of those who are officially recognized as suffering from a disease.

Joan visited three doctors, and each one refused to acknowledge her belief that a common consumer item had caused her sickness. In the absence of a professional diagnosis, Joan constructed her own disease theory. Joan is not simply fabricating an illness narrative to render her somatic troubles meaningful to her; she is also theorizing the etiology and pathophysiology of her sickness and proscribing treatment strategies to reduce the deleterious effects of her sickness. In short, Joan appropriates the language of biomedicine to locate her body in the nomenclature of disease and thus shifts the social location of theorizing disease from physicians to nonphysicians. It is in this fashion that Joan's illness narrative, her subjective experience of distress, begins to sound like a disease narrative, a technical account of the origins, pathways, and treatments of a legitimate biomedical disorder.

Another way of considering this shift is to visualize Joan moving a language from an expert system to a nonexpert system, from the protected sphere of a licensed profession to the more contingent and negotiated sphere of communal life. While this shift may not appear particularly important at first, it gains a measure of significance when it is situated within a defining feature of late modern life: the increasing dependence of ordinary people on abstract or expert systems (Giddens 1990, 1991; Beck 1992). An increasing number of life experiences are created and shaped by technical knowledge that remains abstruse and opaque to most people. Ordinary people who have troubling experiences are likely to seek professional or expert advice. The troubling experience is a biographical moment; the professional or expert offers an explanation of that troubled moment, creating a growing chasm between biographical moments and their subsequent explanations. The person who awakes in a house heated and cooled by electricity, motors, pumps, and thermostats, drives to work in a car with automatic transmission and cruise control, types on a word processor, and sends a message by fax to a client in another country is caught in a tangled web of dependence on expert systems. The abstract technical systems ensnaring her both created these technologies and are required when they break down.

Dependence almost always begs the question of trust, however. And the more dependent we become on abstract systems, the more complicated are the questions of trust (Giddens 1990, 1991). The trust we invest in abstract systems is less a matter of conscious choice between viable alternatives and more, in Anthony Giddens's words, "a tacit acceptance of circumstances in which other alternatives are largely foreclosed" (1990, 90).

When we require expert systems we seek out system representatives, or experts. Experts are the intersections between ordinary people and abstract knowledge systems. In these encounters, according to Giddens, expert systems become vulnerable to skepticism and lose the trust of people whose problems remain in spite of the efforts of the experts. Joan's story suggests a modification of this idea by suggesting that at these intersections the legitimacy of expert systems is less at risk than the credibility of experts. Most people are impatient when an expert representing an abstract system cannot fix a technological trouble. In the event an expert cannot repair a faulty technology, however, people are not likely to abandon the expert system or the hardware it created; rather, they are more likely to desert the expert while retaining their faith in the system.

Abandoning an expert while retaining faith in an abstract system acts to protect the legitimacy of the system. It is the person who represents the system and not the system itself that is rejected. The act of finding another expert expresses a tacit faith in the integrity of the abstract system independent of the skill of this or that expert. Joan's example, however, reveals how people lose trust in a whole class of experts, bypass them, and access the system on their own, in the absence of licensed representation.

Social Definition

It is reasonable to assume that if the environmentally ill are moving away from physician-experts while appropriating the symbols and meanings located in the biomedical-expert system, it is possible to discern the vague outlines of a new way of knowing that links (or relinks) experience with explanation and protests an important accomplishment of the Enlightenment project that successfully separated the two. People who conclude that they are suffering from MCS or EI, who construct theories about the origins of their sickness (its pathophysiology), and conceive of treatment strategies to manage a complicated array of symptoms are claiming the privilege to classify their bodies as *diseased,* not simply ill. If shifting the social location of theorizing the body as diseased from expert to nonexpert systems hints at an alternative way of knowing the world, it does so in large part because of the changes in social definition that accompany this shift. Once expert knowledge is uprooted from its location in expert cultures and placed in communal, nonexpert settings, its logics for apprehending the world might also change.

Rational or technical knowledge does more than describe; it also justifies social and political arrangements (Habermas 1968). Importantly, it promotes a way of knowing that obscures its own social foundations. Rational, particularly scientific, knowledge "conceptualizes an absolute social-natural disconnection" (Wright 1992, 58). By denying its own social commitments, technical knowledge in the hands of experts can pronounce on the affairs of nature and the body as an objective, unbiased witness.

Science is important to the state in its capacity to legitimate a political economy in terms that cannot be easily recognized as social. A product of modernity, biomedicine shares with the major social institutions of the era a remarkable capacity to avoid self-examination. Paraphrasing Gellner, Wright (1992) argues that "genuine knowledge is inherently indifferent" to biography or inequality; it is, rather, "inherently scientific" (50). "Genuine explanation," Gellner writes, "means subsumption under a structure or schema made up of neutral, impersonal elements. In this sense, explanation is always 'dehumanizing,' and inescapably so" (quoted in Wright 1992, 50).

In spite of the popularity of the holistic and community health movements, the importance of scientific assumptions to modern medicine persists. Descartes might be in hiding from the postmodernists, but he is alive and well in the profession of medicine.

> It is a mistake to underestimate the force of Cartesian dualism in medicine today. In spite of a growing disaffection of a section of the populace with traditional approaches to health, the dualist philosophy is alive and well, the guiding light of almost all theoretical and clinical efforts of Western medicine. (Dossey 1984, 13; see also Young 1982; Gordon 1988; Freund and McGuire 1991)

A professor of psychiatry and medicine writes: "The biomedical model embraces both reductionism, the philosophic view that complex phenomena are ultimately derived from a single primary principle, and mind body dualism, the doctrine that separates the mental from the somatic" (Engle 1977, 130).

One observer attributes the tenacity of biomedical assumptions and practices to the continued hegemony of "naturalism" in modern culture. A domain assumption of the Enlightenment, naturalism asserts that humans are a part of nature; they are bio-organic processes that will reveal themselves to those trained in the scientific method (Gordon 1988, 21). The politics of naturalism begins with the capabilities and constraints of the biological body as the sources of individual, social, and economic relationships (Johnstone 1992). To know something from the vantage point of naturalism is to imagine it in its simplest form, uncomplicated by political or economic arrangements. Not surprisingly, the emergence of naturalism corresponded closely with the emergence of the "bourgeois individual," each cultural idea reinforcing the other. The creation story of both early and late modern capitalism "would have to begin with 'In the beginning there was the individual . . .'" (Gordon 1988, 34).

Indeed, the modern period worked to shape the human being as independent of history, "autonomous and thus essentially [a] non-social moral being" (Dumont 1986, 25). The person in modernity was freed from the dead "hand of custom," from the greedy grasp of local traditions; now science and its partner the state would serve to legislate the self (Bauman 1993, 83). Sontag locates the idea of the bourgeois individual in biomedicine, citing Groddeck's eighteenth-century observation that "the sick man himself creates his disease. . . . he is the cause of the disease and we need seek none other" and Karl Menninger's quite similar conclusion reached two hundred years later that "'illness is in part what the world had done to a victim, but in a larger part it is what the victim had done with his world, and with himself'" (quoted in Sontag 1989, 46–47). Consider the painful words of Katherine Mansfield, written in 1923, a year before her death: "A bad day . . . horrible pains go on, and weakness. I could do nothing. The weakness was not only physical. I must heal my self before I will be well. . . . This must be done alone and at once. It is at the root of my not getting better" (quoted in Sontag 1989, 47).

Joining naturalism with the bourgeois individual ensured that the bio-organic person would be considered prior to society and the technical proficiency of biomedicine would be based in part on its claim to mirror the natural, not the social, world. Only by claiming to identify and explain somatic troubles in the absence of politics and history can biomedicine claim its privileged access to natural processes. Physicians, of course, often speak publicly about a health problem, adding their influential voices to important social concerns, but when they do so, they are not speaking from the vantage point of biomedicine. It is the *model* of biomedicine that interests us, not the individual physician.

Apprehending modern problems as biomedical is a potent rhetorical strategy for deflecting attention from the possible social sources of troubles, focusing instead on their supposed biological or psychological origins. Sociology identified this process years ago as "medicalization." Conrad and Schneider (1990), for example, examine the transformation of the "unruly child" into the child with "hyperkinetic impulse disorder" (HID) by tracing the application of biomedical terms to a form of deviant social behavior. Capturing "unruly" children in biomedical language exercised by the profession of medicine divested their aberrant behavior of its cultural and political significance. When the label HID is invoked, the family culture and the political arrangements it reflects are left unexamined as possible sources of a child's anxious behavior. Medicalization expresses the tenacity of naturalism and individualism in contemporary society.

Joan's narrative, however, hints at an alternative strategy for using biomedical language to apprehend a somatic trouble. Joan is not a physician. She is not licensed by the state to capture personal troubles in expert systems. Nevertheless, she appropriates clusters of words from the vocabulary of medicine and in the milieu of her personal and communal world constructs an account of her trouble. Her account begins by externalizing the source of her misery. She is not making herself sick; putatively safe environments and the supposedly safe products found in them are the cause of her sickness. Joan's theory begins with the idea of a well body encountering pathogenic environments. It is not the industrial, polluted environments of the typical contaminated community that are making her sick but the culturally defined safe and nurturing environments of homes and grocery stores. Encoded in Joan's somatic misery and the story she tells about it is the need to invert the normal logic of the sick role, deflecting attention from a clinical appraisal of the physical body to a critical appraisal of the social body. In her hands, EI becomes a lingual representation of a once healthy body protesting imperfections in the production of modern material life.

She theorizes that her sickness is caused by chemicals commonly found in pesticides manufactured for use in houses. Though her exposure to these chemicals occurred in a single incident and was not detected in subsequent blood tests, Joan is certain that her troubles started when she used a bug bomb. Moreover, Joan's theory includes an account of how the chemicals changed her body, rendering it susceptible to violent reactions from minute, subclinical exposures to unrelated chemicals found everywhere in her environment. Her pathophysiology theory keeps the focus on the external environment as the source of her misery. Finally, her treatment strategies suggest the importance of other people in the successful management of her EI. It is useful to think of MCS as a relational disease. That is, it can be successfully managed only if people and environments surrounding the sick person conform to the comparatively austere demands of the illness. Consider the well-chosen words of one woman with a long history of EI:

> More than with any other illness, what other people do or do not do affects those of us with MCS. We are at their mercy. . . . if our spouse insists on smoking, if friends and relatives won't give up their perfumes . . . if hospitals persist in using toxic cleaning products, if restaurants continue putting air "fresheners" in washrooms, . . . and on and on— there's very little we can do. . . . We can only try to protect ourselves.

Unless the person with MCS remains isolated, his or her well-being is directly dependent on the choices and behaviors of others. If people do choose to change their behaviors to accommodate the chemically reactive, they will be motivated in part by plausible, rational explanations of the need for change.

Social Representation

When another person acknowledges the body of the chemically reactive person by making some accommodation to its exacting, some might say extreme, demands, a new body is being socially represented. If MCS signals the emergence of a new body, this body becomes interesting socially and politically only when it finds individuals, organizations, and institutions willing to change their habits, routines, and policies in order to represent it. Joan's somatic trouble in a local grocery store suggests the most basic way the MCS body succeeds in securing representation: it demands it.

Joan told a story about her body, and the store clerk and manager responded to her distress. It is not known whether either person believed Joan's account of her troubles. The manager was probably motivated to assist Joan as much to remove her from his store as to relieve her of her distress, but he did so in a kind way and she appreciated the help. And through his behavior, he momentarily joined Joan in a public drama that acknowledged the reality of a sick body.

The interesting question, however, is not what happened to Joan at a local grocery store but how to, or whether society is prepared to, reorganize to prevent Joan and those like her from becoming sick. If the chemically reactive are going to live among others whose bodies have not changed, they must persuade these others that concepts of disease and environment are now coterminous, with one somehow implying the other. The social and economic costs of succeeding in this rhetorical work are understandably high.

Just how persuasive are laypersons who borrow a medical vernacular to ask others to commit substantial resources to redesign houses, workplaces, public spaces, and so on to represent a strange and troubling body? This hints at the much broader question of how institutions learn. This more abstract question will become clearer if we quickly summarize the ideas of social location and social definition.

The environmentally ill are shifting the traditional location of theorizing by appropriating the language of physician-experts to conceptualize their own somatic misery. In relocating this expert language from its professional setting to the more mundane setting of communal life, the environmentally ill are also challenging a definitional logic of medical expertise that effectively obscures the role of history and politics in the etiology of sickness by identifying the sources of their somatic disorders in the chemical culture of post–World War II America. The third and final question is a pragmatic one: So what? Who is listening and why? It is one thing to borrow a biomedical vernacular and use it to charge society with robbing you of your health while holding it responsible for your recovery; it is quite another to convince influential others that your disease claim is a legitimate one. A new theory of the body in relationship to the environment assumes political relevance if people and institutions are willing to change their behaviors in response to its logics of social culpability and demands for social changes, in spite of the medical profession's steadfast refusal to accept the new theory.

The chemically reactive are in the unenviable position of having to persuade some members of their interpersonal worlds to accept MCS as a legitimate, albeit strange, disease. Persuading others (as we will see) depends in part on the person's ability to manipulate the style and grammar of biomedicine. It is reasonable to assume that the more unusual and exotic the theory of disease and the more it requires unaccustomed changes on the part of family, friends, neighbors, and workmates, the more difficulty a person will have in convincing others of its medical legitimacy. People who accept MCS as a legitimate disorder also acknowledge their responsibility for changing personal habits that might trigger symptoms; they become accountable for both causing and abating disease symptoms. Not everyone in the interpersonal world of the environmentally ill is willing to assume this responsibility. What is striking, however, is just how many are.

Convincing people who occupy the personal spaces of the chemically reactive that ordinary environments are sources of disease might appear to be a considerably different exercise than convincing employers, government agencies, or legislatures to recognize the problem. While there are some differences, both venues require the claimant to present a carefully crafted account of the bioscience etiology of MCS, ensuring that medical nomenclature itself shapes the struggle for consensus. It is in the arenas of work and policy that MCS as a social movement begins to take shape and form.

In summary, if EI constitutes a new way of knowing the body in its relationships to the environment, it is politically important to the extent it changes opinions, social arrangements, and the distribution of resources. Limited to a subjective appraisal that something is wrong with the body's relationship to the environment, even if that appraisal is biomedical in nature, MCS is not likely to be a vehicle for notable social change. On the other hand, as the biomedical appraisal succeeds in convincing influential others that subclinical exposure to ordinary environments is the cause of disease—in spite of the efforts of the medical profession, the chemical and insurance industries, and others to deny the veracity of this claim—it becomes a moral vocabulary that justifies effective action on behalf of the sick. From this vantage point, MCS becomes a cluster of terms that succeed, albeit modestly as of this writing, in redefining the relationship of the body to the built environments of the late twentieth century.

Throughout this book, the idea of EI as a new way of knowing the body in its relationship to built environments is revealed in the activities of ordinary people who claim the right to theorize their bodies and thus shift the social location of theory construction from experts to nonexperts. The contours of this new knowledge become more visible as we record how these theorists change the definitional strategies of science from a focus on nature and the person to a critique of society. Finally, the political efficacy of MCS is measured by its rhetorical power to convince the world that modern bodies and the environments they build are undergoing profound change.

~

Chapters 3 through 5 describe in considerable detail the work accomplished by people forced to comprehend their bodies' rejection of built environments and the commercial products found in them. Our specific interest is in how people learn to think differently about their bodies and the spaces they occupy. In their own words, the chemically reactive describe how they respond to troubling somatic signs and symptoms with reasonable actions that to some degree reduce their miseries. In their practical work to accommodate their selves to their sick bodies, the environmentally ill borrow and change the language of medicine, expanding its explanatory reach to account for a new and troubling disease.

In reading and rereading the narratives of the environmentally ill, we discerned three stages people are likely to go through on their way to theorizing new relationships between their bodies and environments. Perhaps best understood as relatively fixed points in the swirl of narrative materials, these stages are not to be thought of as formal and regimented. Rather, they are simply biographical moments in a person's quest for reasonable explanations, marking a passage from one stage in this journey to another.

Part Two

Part Two

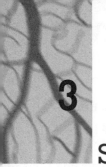

3

Something Unusual
Is Happening Here

Everyone who is born holds dual citizenship, in the
kingdom of the well and in the kingdom of the sick.
Although we all prefer to use only the good passport,
sooner or later each of us is obliged ... to identify
ourselves as citizens of that other place.

(Sontag 1989, 3)

OUR BODIES ARE SURROUNDED by environments and themselves constitute parts of environments that other bodies experience.
In spite of this close affinity with biophysical environments (or, perhaps, because of it), most people do not pay close attention to their
bodies' complex relationships to biospheres and the things in them. In
the absence of obviously dangerous environments that pose immediate threats to survival or physical well-being, the stance taken toward
biophysical surroundings is probably one of "nothing unusual is
going on here." And more likely than not this stance is taken in the
absence of any serious reflection. It is simply assumed, a taken-for-
granted part of what everyone accepts without discussion or proof.

When a woman walks into her backyard or a friend's house, plays
a round of golf, or visits a coffee shop, she is likely to do so without
pausing to ponder the implications of these spaces for her immediate

well-being. Moreover, she can and will assume that her friends, acquaintances, and even strangers experience these spaces as she does; that is, they assume the relative safety of these spaces without requiring tests or proof of their assumptions. There is what Alfred Schutz (1967) calls a "reciprocity of perspectives" regarding our attitude toward routine environments: you and I see, smell, and hear basically the same things and, importantly, our somatic responses to these things will be similar. We are alike and understand each other insofar as each of us takes for granted the routine, predictable quality of our everyday environments. Sustaining social life depends in part on these tacit agreements.

Safe, or nonextreme, environments exist when physical places are embedded in legitimate ways of knowing that render them innocuous and inoffensive. Nonextreme environments are apprehended in an "as if" manner. Indeed, most people, most of the time, act toward their physical environments "as if" they are not dangerous; they do so, in part, because people around them are also acting "as if" the environment is safe (Kroll-Smith 1995). "As if" forms of consciousness are essential for the development of more complex social relationships (Berger and Luckmann 1966; Schutz 1967; Giddens 1991; Kroll-Smith 1995). They are prelinguistic, emotively apprehended contracts between participants that the world enjoys sufficient order to proceed with the tasks at hand. An apropos image of a routine, nonextreme environment is a physical, organic space in which probabilities are not randomly distributed, in which some events are more likely to happen than others and still other events are unlikely to happen at all.

It is true, of course, that not all environments are apprehended prereflectively. Some require imagination or active understanding to comprehend. All societies know this fact and most prepare for it. Sometimes natural weather patterns, or human ignorance, or malfeasance creates dangerous or extreme environments. News reporting regularly features accounts of such dangerous environments as tornadoes and hurricanes, or toxic waste sites and radioactive fallout. Few people would debate whether these types of environments are risks to personal and collective well-being. Most modern societies learn to anticipate these dangers, however, and develop (more or less) coordinated city, state, and federal responses to them.

Societies and the bodies that inhabit them are thus organized to reflect a general consensus regarding safe and dangerous places (Durkheim 1965; Douglas 1966). The areal distribution of these places is an accepted part of what everybody knows about environments. Violating the reciprocity of perspectives regarding the demarcations between routine and dangerous environments are a growing number of people who believe their bodies are reacting violently and unexpectedly to physical places acknowledged as benign, if not nurturing. Central to MCS is its premise that bodies are made sick by these putatively clean spaces; they simply cannot withstand them.

In these culturally defined safe spaces where an ordinary body exists free from danger and hurt, an environmentally ill body is more likely to call attention to itself as an obstacle to routine social exchange, raising the disturbing question Why is this body different from ours? A more disturbing question follows: Is he or she human like us? In some respects those with MCS are in a struggle to be accepted as human. To do so, they must shift attention from an exclusive focus on their bodies to a careful reconsideration of what are acknowledged as safe, clean places. The resistance they face is based in part on the social and political changes that must follow if the bodies of the chemically reactive are acknowledged as real.

The environmentally ill recall how their bodies were initially thrown off balance and how they first tried to sustain "a nothing unusual is happening here stance." When commonsense, or "what everybody knows," explanations fail to account for all of their somatic changes, however, they admit their bodies can no longer be taken for granted; rather, they must be thought about, pondered, and mused over. It is the first change in a series of changes that culminate in people developing new theories about their bodies and the routine, nonextreme places they occupy. And it is a change that few of the environmentally ill forget. If narration is a process in which the self is joined to a new definition of the body and its relationship to environments, then we are not surprised to learn that 80 percent of respondents in a nonrandom survey of sixty-eight hundred chemically reactive people claimed to know "when, where, with what, and how they were made ill" (quoted in Ashford and Miller 1991, 5).

Entering the EI Career

The process of becoming aware that something unusual is happening to the body and its relationship to the environment begins, somewhat ironically, with recognizing that something unpleasant or downright disagreeable, but not unexpected, has occurred. This process takes one of two forms: through an acute exposure to a chemical agent or agents and the immediate association of signs and symptoms accompanying the exposure; or through a simple recognition that unpleasant changes in the body are occurring with no immediate recognition that they are caused by local environments.

Acute Exposure

A professional musician describes her place of employment, an opera house that is a completely sealed environment:

> The hydraulic which raises and lowers the pit malfunctioned, spewing fumes into the pit through its air-intake plenums. . . . I began to get respiratory infections regularly. . . . later in the season I was exposed to formaldehyde offgassing from large quantities of raw plywood in a recording studio. These exposures were the origins of my MCS.

Several of her fellow musicians also experienced problems caused by the initial exposures in the orchestra pit. Indeed, there is nothing surprising in people getting sick when they are exposed to excessive amounts of hydraulic fluids and formaldehyde. Her colleagues, however, recovered. She did not.

A government employee was exposed to a "toxic cocktail" while working as an inspector for a state department of environmental resources. He was responding to a complaint from residents who smelled caustic odors coming from an abandoned used car lot in their neighborhood. He provides the following account of his exposure:

> I'm the only one who suggested we needed samples. Like digging into the ground. I didn't bring sampling equipment. Besides, soil sampling was not part of my job at the DER. Some state troopers loaned us shovels and someone found some jars. The emergency response guy dug and I pointed. We were all greatly relieved to find something. . . . We started smelling strange things coming from the ground. At that point, the state police should have pulled us back. No one was wearing a respirator. But everyone was so excited that we finally found something out there, that we proceeded on our merry way. The bigger the smells were, you know, that was pay dirt. We had this guy digging. I was just following my nose, smelling, stopping, pointing, and someone would dig. I was like a hunting dog.
>
> Once we collected the samples, and the excitement of the big discovery was not so exciting, I noticed the smells burning my nose, eyes, my throat, my skin, and such. And it was a strange feeling. The guy with the shovel had to call me a couple of times, because apparently I was in the rapture of the deep, kind of like I had crawled into a big shell and couldn't hear the world. If you've ever scuba dived, I did several years ago, it was like having nitrogen narcosis. I was giddy and losing my balance.

How did this man interpret his unsavory experience? Quite simply as an "occupational hazard." "It happens in work like mine," he reasoned.

A graduate student who suffers from MCS remembers her acute exposure:

> My disability began after I was "crop-dusted" twenty-two years ago. . . . Although I became ill the same day that I was sprayed . . . I did not connect the spraying with my illness until much later. The pilot had opened the valve before getting to the field. I didn't think that I received

much exposure and I was naive and not afraid of chemicals, and in fact never thought to tell my physician at the time about the incident. At the time, I believed in "better living through chemistry."

For this woman and others who enter the EI career through an acute exposure, there is, in retrospect, little doubt about the origin of their troubles, but there is little surprise or occasion for wonder. "Accidents happen. Things can go wrong. I understand all that," reasoned a man who was sprayed with malathion while working in a city pest control project. A city sewerage employee contaminated in a chlorine spill explained her unexpected exposure by invoking a modern wisdom: "Shit happens."

In these and related accounts, people who later identify themselves as environmentally ill normalize their initial and sudden chemical insults, placing them in the category of what everybody knows: accidents happen, and while they are unfortunate, they are not necessarily unusual. At this stage in becoming chemically reactive, it is not necessary to construct a novel way of knowing the body and its relationship to the environment. Instead of a new practical epistemology, the old one will do just fine, to wit, bad things sometimes happen to good people. In addition, biomedicine is prepared to identify and explain somatic responses to acute exposures. Symptom lists are matched with chemical agents, treatment strategies are common lore and routinely work. Moreover, toxicology will predict that most people commonly recover from an acute exposure with no lasting or residual effects (Ashford and Miller 1991).

Chronic Exposure

A retired teacher recounts a series of ordinary, unexceptional activities and events she believes are the sources of her illness:

> We lived in a rural mountain village with clean air. . . . We gardened organically . . . backpacked and exercised. . . . I knew nothing about formaldehyde. Urea formaldehyde foam insulation was blown into the house we rented in 1979. We lived there until 1987 when we moved

into an eight-year-old double-wide mobile home which we painted inside and out. I taught in a brand-new carpeted classroom. In 1984 my classroom was insulated with styrofoam on the interior walls. I took two different antibiotics in 1987 for a stubborn hand infection. . . . I refinished many pieces of furniture for our home and my classroom. I silk-screened for many years. My symptoms developed gradually over nine years until November of 1988. Two students led me to the office at noon and I never returned to work.

Alice remembers:

About 1975, whatever year Hurricane Frederick came through our area, the office area of our retail electronics store had to be relocated due to damage. Our entire operation was temporarily relocated, but I worked mainly in the office. My office was in the work area of a former tire store. . . . I experienced very dry nasal passages and some eye discomfort the entire time we were located there.

Sometime after this, we bought a lot and my husband put sulphur powder on his pants legs to keep the red bugs off. I had a rather severe reaction to the sulphur powder. I washed his clothes with some of mine and had to wash mine about ten times before I was able to purge them from the sulphur powder enough to wear them and not prickle all over and have a very dry nose.

We had blueprints drawn up and, when going over them to check for changes after they were printed, I thought I was taking a cold for several days—slightly sore throat, fatigue, stuffy nose, and scratchy eyes.

We then built a new home with a basement which was located about five hundred feet from a golf course. . . . my condition steadily worsened. Thinking I had an allergy, my family doctor sent me to a very good allergy group which diagnosed the problem as . . . a vasomotor reaction.

A legal secretary writes:

I started working for a lawyer. He had just completed major renovations on a new office . . . the smell was very strong. I . . . lost my job in

1990 when I grew increasingly ill, was unable to eat, and lost thirty pounds. . . . I was hospitalized twice, the first time for two weeks, on intravenous feedings and the second time for four days to have a specialist try to determine what was wrong. At that time Crohn's disease was suspected.

A dentist recalls

seeing my first patient at 8 A.M. and being ready to go to back to sleep at 9. I thought at first I had yuppie disease, you know chronic fatigue. I couldn't think clearly and was irritated for no apparent reason. Again, I attributed this to chronic fatigue syndrome. But then some really bizarre things started. My joints started to swell, painfully, and I had diarrhea about every other day. I started to lose weight and noticed my skin bruising when I bumped into something. I could even bruise myself by pressing my thumb on my arm. . . . I started to feel like something was in my body, and it wasn't me, like that girl in *The Exorcist*.

Although acute and gradual entrées into MCS differ markedly from one another, both are likely to be explained initially using various commonsense or "everybody knows" accounts. Everybody knows, for example, that allergies run in families and that toxic chemicals are to be avoided. In this fashion, something problematic is absorbed into something taken for granted. Crohn's disease is a recognized, if unfortunate, medical condition. And while no one wants to be possessed by the devil, possession is a known—if not necessarily believed in—cultural phenomenon. Karen started her MCS career by noticing small changes in her body, including a loss of energy, stiff joints, and allergy-like symptoms. She brought these signs to the attention of her mother, who explained that allergies "run in the family" and that fatigue and stiffness could mean Karen had a "cold in her body," drawing a distinction between such a cold and one that was in her head. Temporarily satisfied with her mother's explanation of her symptoms, Karen adopted a casual attitude toward her somatic troubles. If these conventional or commonsense explanations rendered an account of the problem sufficient to treat it and move on, our story would end here. The bodies in question, however, resist routine attempts to classify and treat them.

Acute- and gradual-onset cases begin to merge into one class of trouble as people become aware of some kind of connection between their symptoms and the ordinary environments they encounter every day. At this juncture a shift from "nothing unusual is happening here" to "something out of the ordinary is occurring" is made. Consider Elliot's story.

> I was an industrial painter living in Los Angeles. For over seven years I worked fifty hours a week painting the insides of factories, threaders, rollers, line equipment, and so on. I am thirty-two years old and enjoyed good health until about a year ago when I began noticing some weird things. While driving to work one morning my shoulder and neck muscles began to jerk around. I almost lost control of the car. I also began to forget things about this time. I would forget why I was in a store, what I was supposed to buy, the time of day and sometimes the day of the week. I would forget these things. Once I forgot my phone number. Then there was the nausea and skin rashes. I also had trouble breathing. I noticed my problems were worse when I went to work.
>
> I made an appointment with an internist to get a checkup. This is weird. I am standing behind a woman who is paying her bill in the doctor's office. I rested my hand against the wall, just leaning on it waiting my turn. When I pulled my hand down from the wall I had paint all over it and there was a spot on the wall that looked just like my hand. I thought the wall had just been painted.

In fact the wall had not been painted for years. Later clinical studies would show that industrial paint solvent emitted from Elliot's sweaty palm literally took the paint off the wall. The concentration of industrial-strength solvents in his bloodstream required several days of detoxification to clean out. Although Elliot was pronounced clean of industrial chemicals and found a less noxious job as a construction worker, he continued to experience his original symptoms with increasing severity. He was increasingly anxious over his apparent sensitivity to ordinary synthetic materials and some foods, sources of physical distress unrelated to the chemicals in the paint solvents. After missing several days of work because of weakness, headaches, trembling, and other unusual symptoms, he filed a workers' compensation claim against his former employer.

Elliot is now building a ceramic house trailer because he has become too reactive to the environments in his apartment, neighborhood, and community. He plans to move his finished trailer to the Sierra Madres, hoping to find relief from his symptoms in the more rarefied mountain air.

Karen, who started with allergy symptoms and a "body cold," soon found she was "going brain dead" and was unable to stop itching. Moreover, like Elliot, she experienced her symptoms increasing and decreasing in severity in relationship to the environments she was in. In her account of what she calls her "wake-up call that something was not right there," she describes putting on a new raincoat, a birthday gift from her parents. "I no sooner had my arms in that coat than I started to get a rash. . . . I tore it off and ran to the bathroom and ran cold water on my arms. I was sick the rest of the day. . . . My mother tried the coat on and she was fine. . . . I later learned that it was weatherproofed with some chemical I react to."

Ann, who was exposed to agricultural pesticides for several years, suffered from chronic bronchitis, which she attributed to the pesticides. While many physicians and toxicologists would argue that her exposure to pesticides was well below levels considered dangerous to human health, there is nevertheless a known relationship between respiratory diseases and pesticides (Duehring and Wilson 1994, 10). In the following account Ann describes how she became aware that something out of the ordinary was happening to her, something more quixotic and horrifying than bronchitis.

In March 1991, I was out in the garage for a considerable length of time with the doors shut as it was foggy and cold, when I suddenly came down with sensations of being electrocuted up and down my spine. My arms were also being electrocuted and my whole body vibrated. My arms became semiparalyzed and every joint made popping sounds. . . . When I shut my eyes I saw black and white spots like a scrambled TV screen or geometric patterns. The pain felt like I was being eaten alive.

A former chemical engineer remembers:

In the summer of 1984, I had been working for three months in their specialty chemical division. I began to get chest pains if I inhaled small quantities of isocyanates or drank coffee. I went to see a doctor, who explained that I should be careful. I was not aware of my poor thinking, for on December 14, 1984, I instructed a machine operator to add methanol to a drum of toluene diisocyanate. . . . Of course there was an exothermic reaction and the liquid TDI burped out of the drum. I helped clean up the spill. My memory is poor about the cleanup. . . . I remember 3M's lawyers making a mockery of my memory in the workers' compensation hearing. The next morning after the spill, I experienced chest pains in my home that I associated with inhaling small quantities of isocyanates. During the next month, I recognized painful symptoms from more and more objects, but I was totally unaware what had happened. I mistakenly thought that I had brought TDI home on my clothes. The more I did the more I seemed to be in pain. I started to react to mold, fabric softener, perfumes, most detergents, chemical fertilizers, glycols, and lots of other chemicals. If these things are present in a room I am in pain.

Betty, a chemist, recalls in rather graphic terms her realization that something terrible was happening to her body:

I would have shortness of breath and irregular heartbeat. . . . the skin on the inside of my right nostril would peel off. I had muscle spasms, "tics," and seizurelike activity. . . . I had uterine contractions for six hours (like labor). Within ten days my uterine wall fell off in one sheet. . . . I began to have breathing problems after taking certain medications. . . . I was exposed to the chemical ethylene oxide over a ten-year period. From 1980 until 1984 I had daily (five days a week) high-level exposures, due to a gas sterilizer exhausting the entire load into the working area.

Betty believed there was an association between her exposure to ethylene oxide and her physical deterioration.

A recreational dancer describes a series of unsuccessful efforts to hold a job as her body became increasingly unmanageable:

> Unaware that smoke is an EI patient's major problem next to perfume in public places, I ballroom danced in smoke-filled bars. I began to experience memory loss and would not know where I was at on the dance floor. . . . At my job I worked with carbonless files and felt myself heating up inside as if a match were burning me. I would have brain fog and confusion, and at one point did not know what to do with a bundle of papers that I signed on a daily basis. . . . I often cried and made so many mistakes I lost my job. I tried to work in retail, but had such brain fog when handling money and objects that I caught myself handing a customer the change that she owed me. The drawer had been missing money and . . . I had blamed my supervisor. It was clear to me, however, that I had been handing money out to customers. I ended up losing that job as well. At . . . another job, I worked less than two hours with checks at a processing center; the ink from the machine made the inside of my head swell up so badly that I became emotional and started to cry. I lost that job as well.

The transition in this first stage is from the initial experience of symptoms as perhaps unfortunate and distressing but not particularly unusual, to apprehending the body as acting strange and unpredictable in what were once routine and putatively safe environments. Norman Denzin (1993) captures the anxiety of this transition in his concept of the "epiphanal moment," a liminal period wherein the person is betwixt and between "interpretive frameworks" (91). Reflecting on that moment at the onset of her illness when she was without the words to interpret her symptoms, a woman with EI recalls, "I thought I wasn't human."

These accounts provide stories of bodies that become increasingly disorderly in mundane, putatively safe places—garages, offices, workshops, or houses—and bodies that react unexpectedly to common consumer items. Interpreting these narratives as statements about environments, it is possible to discern a transformation or change in the definitions of safe and dangerous places. What was once safe is now dangerous or extreme.

The Random House College Dictionary defines *extreme* as a condition or state farthest removed from the ordinary. Something is considered ordinary if it can be apprehended and responded to in a routine manner; that same thing might be experienced as extreme if it eludes efforts at normalization. The idea of extreme suggests the absence of a meaningful way of comprehending an event, a circumstance, or perhaps, as in this case, a place, that produces the (possibly) negative effect of rendering a situation incoherent. Applied to environments, we might say that extreme environments are physical or spatial states that escape or elude common or expert knowledge and therefore are experienced by people as essential puzzlements or profound uncertainties.

In extreme situations, *"as if"* environments are transformed into *"what if?"* environments. Based on the preceding accounts, for example, we can imagine the following reminiscence: "I once thought of my garage [house, backyard, living room, and so on] as if it were a safe place to be. What, in fact, if it is dangerous?" What makes an environment extreme is the joining of a diminishing fund of applicable knowledge with a drastic increase in tension between a person's body and its immediate environments. It is the coincidence of a depreciated fund of useful knowledge with an amplified awareness of the need to respond that characterizes the extreme environment. Thus, an environment may be said to be extreme when it narrows the range of what people know about their somatic relationships to physical places and things while simultaneously intensifying their need to respond to their bodies and their material surroundings with imperfect knowledge. Extreme environments mark a momentary or extended period of ontological insecurity; physical circumstances of place are now uncertain, and traditional coping strategies are increasingly ineffective.

Perhaps it is not particularly useful for most of us to consider causal direction at those moments when physical states mirror ideal meanings. But when bodies and environments are incoherent and conventional meanings no longer make sense, people are apt to conceptualize their somatic and environmental distress, theorizing their misery in a manner that allows them to understand and manage it. Environmental illness is a theory of the body and the environment constructed of necessity, driven by discomfort and pain. It joins a mind to a body that is no longer readily intelligible by cobbling together clusters of words to tell a story of disease.

If sick bodies are organizing thoughts, as we propose, it is worth pausing to assay these bodies as they are experienced by the persons who inhabit them. Consider the following several descriptions of sick bodies offered by people who would later interpret themselves as environmentally ill.

A "partially disabled building contractor" writes:

> My body becomes my worst nightmare. I feel like Freddie [from the movie *Nightmare on Elm Street*] lives inside me. I start to drool uncontrollably. I get confused . . . forgetting where I am. I feel electrical shocks inside my skin. I want to scratch my skin off, but it hurts too much to touch it. Sometimes I just cry and my fingernails turn blue. My tongue gets thick and rolls around in my mouth like a big piece of fat. Eating makes me gag. I want to sleep but I'm too nervous.

A retired program analyst for the Department of Defense describes her body as

> Itching and burning. With headache, chills, sweats, numbness, and swelling in my hands, pain along my right arm and in the ball of my left foot, gastrointestinal problems (nausea, dysentery, . . . constipation),

feeling of being drugged, nasal stuffiness, agitation, weakness, lethargy (body-like-lead syndrome, in which I weigh three hundred pounds instead of the one hundred I actually weigh), hoarseness, thick-feeling tongue and difficulty speaking, cough, irritability, confusion, depression.

A former products engineer borrows from biology to describe his body: "My ears itch and I get excessive mucus in my mouth, almost gagging me. My neck gets a tick jerking me back and forth. I swell up like a balloon and I get pimples. Pimples! I'm forty-one years old. Maybe I'm de-evolving, or regressing. I feel like a mutating cell."

A former insurance agent sums up his body:

> I have this general feeling I am going to die. . . . My family is getting intolerant with me. . . . I woke up yesterday and my eyelids were swollen and cracked and my feet were numb. I tried to tell my boy how bad I felt and my tongue just kept getting bigger, or I felt like it did. I couldn't say my words. It was like someone stuffed a bunch of marbles in my mouth.

A housewife laughs quietly as she attributes to her body a capacity for intentional behavior:

> I was thinking the other day that my body had become my enemy. Like it wants to hurt me. Like it says, "*Ahh,* today I'm going to wheeze, swell up, cramp, get real anxious and sweat profusely. . . . I know I'm talking like this isn't my body, but it isn't. . . . You asked me what my body feels like? I'll tell you what it feels like, like a nightmare. So there.

A former college administrator imagines her body as

> a creature likely to be found in a Grimm fairy tale. Yeah, I have become a monstrous fable. When I go somewhere I wonder do people see me as hideous. . . . when I get up in the morning I don't want to look in a mirror. I am afraid of the grotesque thing that will stare back at me. The funny thing is, though, I look normal.

An environmental activist specializing in "safe schools" often feels like her body is "being held hostage by a hostile synthetic environment. . . . I am less resilient to my environment. . . . Having this illness is like living in a body infested with dandelions. I never know where or when the next group of weeds will sprout."

A professional musician imagines

> being in a wheelchair, and there were barriers everywhere. You couldn't walk up to a person, without a tree in the way (their fragrance). You couldn't get out your door, because of pesticide barriers. . . . Ramps don't mean anything, the chemical barriers are far worse than the physical barriers.

Finally, a college professor describes her illness and body by asking the reader to imagine his or her body as if it were incarcerated:

> Imagine that suddenly you must spend your life in prison, but the prison is something you always carry with you, like a turtle carries its shell. If you slip out between the bars, if you escape, you will meet the equivalent of an electrified fence: excruciating pain. . . . And what keeps you locked up, robbed of the freedom you once experienced as natural as your own breath? It is what you breathe, what has been spewed into the natural air, unregulated chemicals from almost everywhere. . . . Imagine that every step you take is over a minefield, that at any moment something which doesn't affect most others . . . will explode in your face. . . . Imagine that you carry your own prison but no one but you sees the bars.

A striking feature of these accounts is their remarkable thoughtfulness. Thick descriptions, enhanced by the clever use of analogies, suggest the environmentally ill body has become a mysterious and ambiguous thing. Fairy tales, genetics, horticulture, law enforcement, war, horror films, and nightmares are among the analogies used to convey to the self and others an understanding of this untoward and unpredictable body. An otherwise obscure environmentally ill body becomes intelligible when imagined as a field of weeds or a minefield, as a nightmare, a fabled monster, and so on.

If the environmentally ill simply trafficked in literary symbols to describe their bodies, however, as provocative as such descriptions are, their miseries would invite comparison with Kafka's miserable Gregor Samsa, who

> woke up one morning from unsettling dreams [and] found himself changed in his bed into a monstrous vermin. He was lying on his back as hard as armor plate, and when he lifted his head a little, he saw a vaunted brown belly. . . . His many legs, pitifully thin compared with the size of the rest of him, were waving helplessly before his eyes. (1972, 3)

As Kafka's story unfolds, one is likely to be struck by the absence of any inquiry by Gregor or his family to determine just what turned him into a cockroach and how to turn him back into a human being. His wretched condition was simply accepted and adapted to, though, one might conclude, with rather disappointing results.[1]

Unlike Gregor, the environmentally ill do not simply accept the changes in their bodies, adapting by moving furniture about and changing their diets. Perhaps to escape the fate of those with no plausible stories to represent and explain their misshapen lives or bodies, they construct accounts of their somatic miseries in what Touraine (1995), Beck (1992, 1995), and others (see Giddens 1990) would call the common language of modernity: instrumental rationality.

In this initial stage, people become aware of their bodies turning into something they do not understand. Something indeed unusual is happening to them. Moreover, commonsense accounts of their somatic troubles no longer help them understand the changes in their bodies. If consciousness is shaped in part by the constraints of our bodies, the bodies we have just encountered are likely to encourage a new way of knowing the physical self and its relationship to local environments.

A new way of knowing bodies and their relationships to environments begins, appropriately enough, in the mundane work of reclassification and correlation. If EI is a practical epistemology, it must know something new about the links between somatic troubles and physical spaces. The next chapter examines the process of reclassifying bodies and the material world, and, as a consequence, how the bodies of the chemically reactive stand against biomedical theory.

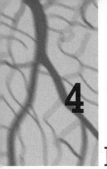

4
Bodies against Theory

What has been called the "search for knowledge"
might be better and more modestly regarded as a
dialogue — among ourselves, and between ourselves and
nature — from which we learn whatever aspects of nature
and ourselves we may need to know in order to go on
surviving.

(Bickerton 1990, 231)

A STRIKING FEATURE of the interviews we collected was the common activities among people who would later identify themselves as chemically reactive. Like sleuths in search of clues, these people interrogate their material environments as possible perpetrators of disease. In systematic fashion they look for relationships between symptoms and specific places and things. Truth for those with MCS is not sought outside of a rational practice.

If the initial stage of EI is accepting the unsettling idea that formerly safe and nurturing places are now health hazards, the second move a chemically reactive person is likely to make is a calculated reassessment of the boundaries between what must now be considered dangerous and what can be approached as safe. In identifying environments that cause sickness and classifying specific symptoms with specific consumer products and chemicals, the environmentally ill organize both their thinking and their routines, creating the possibility of coexisting in a world that has now become a much more dangerous proposition.

A graduate student majoring in business administration recalls:

> I am an orderly person and did not want to panic when I started to get sick from what seemed like everything. I remember walking around my apartment coaching myself to get a grip. . . . I found a legal pad and started to list things that seemed to make me sick and how I would get sick, like hives, joint pain, indigestion, things like that.

A legal secretary imagined her body was "a Geiger counter and I listened for a tick, tick, tick when it got near something it reacted to." A retired dentist recalls becoming "a student of my body. Like I said, 'Okay Mr. body, you me tell what I need to do,' you know, to protect myself." Lynn Lawson, a professional writer, developed what she calls "Lawson's Second Law: You have to be your own personal environmental protection agency. . . . You have to learn how to protect yourself" (1993, 318).

In addition to establishing correlations between places, things, and their bodies, many people also associate specific types of reactions with specific environments and consumer products. Recalling her initial experiences of various changes in her body in relationship to specific places and chemical products, a massage therapist writes:

> I walked into a church basement and started feeling spacey. My balance was affected and my gait changed. A friend helped me get out. When I hit the fresh air, I started crying. After five to ten minutes of fresh air, the crying was under control, but I experienced fatigue and a deflated mood.
>
> An old oil tank was removed from my house. In the process, oil fumes were released into the air and some oil was spilled onto the cement floor. I spent the week climbing the walls, feeling like my seams were fraying on the inside. This reminded me of when I lived near an oil refinery. Whenever I went outside, I felt the same way. At that time, I

didn't understand what was happening and called it "anxiety." This time, when the tank was removed, I knew why I felt the way I did.

I had a mole removed from my face. A local anesthetic was used. Fatigue, depressed mood, digestive disturbances, and dizziness hounded me for several days. Five days later, when the stitches were removed, the doctor kept an isopropyl alcohol-soaked pad on the area. . . . This brought on a crying spell. Several hours later, I went to the emergency room with severe left-side chest pain involving my left arm. . . . Tests showed no lung or heart involvement. . . . I consider this to have been a delayed reaction to the alcohol exposure.

These accounts illustrate both a product of thought, a nascent theory of the body and its relationship to the environment, and a process of thinking. The product and the process, of course, are not unrelated. We examine them both in this chapter, attending first to the process of thinking. Thinking typically proceeds on the basis of at least a few unstated assumptions about how knowing is possible. At the risk of seeming to read too much into the illness narratives, we identify some of the premises that structure the way the chemically reactive approach the problem of theorizing their bodies. Next, several accounts from the chemically reactive tell a remarkable story about causal relationships between recalcitrant and disorderly bodies and the specific environments and consumer products they encounter.

Experiences, Bodies, and the Return of the Subject

What can be said about the process of theorizing EI thus far? The accounts already cited in this chapter and those to come imply a simple but significant observation: a baseline premise for theorizing MCS is a belief that human experience is a valid way of knowing. This premise might strike many readers as lacking in imagination. But it assumes considerable importance when we remember that, in Beck's words, "experience—understood as the individual's sensory understanding of the world—is the orphan child of the scientized world"

(1995, 15). Valid and reliable knowledge in the modern world is the product of experimental science and, pointedly, not subjective experience. People, of course, can trust their senses as sources of knowing; when they do so, however, they cannot claim to know something scientific or medical about themselves or their world. To refer to an observation or thought as subjective is to remove it from serious consideration as a source of expert knowledge. As a theory of disease, however, MCS begins with experiences that oppose biomedical theory. It is almost as if the chemically reactive body is organized against medical science, a body against theory, as it were.

Interpreting the importance of somatic experience to the chemically reactive begins with a simple observation: they do not approach their dilemmas as poststructuralists, assuming their somatic states are products of diverse discourses, symbols that become things. Rather, they pursue an explanation of their sick bodies in the language of naturalism. Like Kenneth Burke's black holes, EI is what it is as it is; it merely has to be empirically identified (1989, 60).

Furthermore, people who experience changes in their bodies' capacities to exist in common and customary settings believe their bodies exist independently of themselves as thinking beings.[1] An electrician in a sewerage treatment plant is challenged by his disease: "I've always been one to figure things out. Now I'm trying to figure my body out, like we're playing a game of chess. . . . Today I'm winning but I might be losing tomorrow." A former dentist recalls his first several months of living with EI: "I kept saying to myself, 'You're not crazy. You are blessed with a good mind. Figure this thing out.' I said something like this to myself every day." "Like everybody, I took my body for granted," remembers a hair stylist; then "it was like my body became this big old Rubic's Cube, a puzzle I was determined to solve." Distancing herself from her illness to gain some control over it, a woman with a degree in psychology writes, "I do not identify myself as chemically sensitive—my body is chemically sensitive and that identifies me!"

While Bryan Turner (1984) can end his lengthy and important

inquiry into the body by admitting that in writing it he has "become increasingly less sure of what the body is" (7), a person whose body is responding in extreme and unexpected ways to what were once known as safe places must be sure of how the body works, what makes it sick, and what makes it well. Most of us are aware of a distinction between our selves and our bodies. For the chemically reactive, however, acknowledging the distance is a first step toward thinking deliberately about their bodies.

Finally, people with EI experience their bodies as sources of unmediated knowledge; importantly, they act toward that knowledge as if it were rational, that is, legitimate. A person can know his self, as opposed to his body, as Mead (1967) reminds us, only "indirectly, from the particular standpoints of other individual members of the same social group or from the generalized standpoint of the social group as a whole to which" he belongs (202). The immediate experience of the body, however, is direct, requiring only consciousness to be real. Our first-order relationship to our bodies, in other words, occurs in the absence of significant social symbols; it is a sensory relationship above all. Somatic pain or pleasure does not require the immediate ratification of others. What typically does require confirmation, however, is how a particular somatic experience is classified and explained. Aggregating, classifying, and explaining bodies has long been recognized by the modern state as an important exercise in control. Foucault (1973) thought it the most penetrating form of modern control and located its most incisive expression in the emergence of medical science. He identified "a spontaneous and deeply rooted convergence between the requirements of political ideology and those of medical technology" (38). The more sophisticated medical technology becomes, the less necessary it is to listen to the person whose body requires attention.

The erosion of the subject in the professional practice of medicine is neatly captured in the now standard social science distinction between illness and disease. "Disease," according to a standard textbook in medical sociology, "refers to a medical concept of pathology

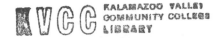

. . . clinically defined by the medical profession." Illness, on the other hand, is the experience of "health and ill-health and is indicated by the person's reactions to the symptoms" (Bond and Bond 1986, 200). The authority to medically evaluate a body and pronounce it diseased is strictly limited to a group of licensed practitioners. In spite of the authority of the medical profession to legislate disease as if there was a body but no person, a diseased body is animated by a subject. While this fact might irritate some physicians, it was an open invitation to social and behavioral scientists. Subjects, it was decided, would experience their diseases as illness behaviors and perceptions, topics ideally suited to the human sciences. In short, while bodies would have diseases, subjects would have illnesses.

This neat separation of the subject from the body renders the personal experiences of bodies unsuitable for biomedical theories. And to be sure, separating bodies from persons is by no means universally decried. To the contrary, it is reasonable to assume that laypersons would not ordinarily dissent from a practice that renders them, simply, bodies if such a practice, however distasteful, results in a cure.

Most people in the second stage of MCS—those who are struggling to identify, classify, and reorder their bodies in relationship to places and things—are also seeing physicians. Among their first moves when they realized that something unusual was happening to them was to seek medical attention. With few exceptions, however, the diagnoses and treatments are not working. Indeed, as we will see in the next chapter, medical treatment often intensifies distress rather than relieving it.

But the important point here is the simultaneous activities of the chemically reactive who are both visiting physicians and working independently of them to determine the causes of their discomfort. People in the nascent stages of MCS often tell their physicians stories about the strange reactions of their bodies when exposed to a seemingly endless array of environments and consumer products. Most doctors, however, cannot affirm the bizarre, queer stories they are told. They are more likely to act like good doctors who try to fit the diagnostic signs they are observing into some recognized disorder, thus routinizing what at first glance is likely to appear anything but routine.

A former hair stylist provides this account:

> I wanted my doctor to tell me what was wrong. To prescribe something and get me well again. But all of the things he called my problem, "adult-onset asthma," "possibly Epstein-Barr," and things didn't help. . . . so I kept worrying, testing my body, like I would say to myself, "Okay, now you are going to walk down the dog food aisle in the grocery store and you're going to see how you feel." I planned to walk down every aisle of our grocery store one weekend and write down how I felt. I only made it down three aisles, though, before I got too sick. My husband thought I was crazy. He told me it wasn't a very good test because if I was reacting to anything (in one aisle) it would be jumbled up with something else (in another aisle). . . . My next plan was to go down one aisle a day and keep a diary of my reactions.

A disabled seamstress writes:

> I had chest constriction. Blood oxygen dropped to 50. The treating physician swore I had a blood clot in my lung. Or heart disease. Guess what? No evidence of any of these. It was a chemical reaction, I told him, but he told me it wasn't. He couldn't figure it out.

A college professor recalls his early visits to his family doctor:

> It got to be a ritual. Every time I sat on his examining table, I would tell him that I thought this or that was making me sick. He would look puzzled, shake his head, and tell me I looked fine. I would tell him I might look fine but I feel terrible. He would tell me the tests were negative. I respond with, "Well, we need to make up some new tests." Both of us thought my symptoms were strange. The difference is I believed what I had was real and he wasn't sure he believed me.

Perhaps his physician couldn't believe. If every way of seeing is also a way of not seeing, biomedicine is an explanation that stops well short of an inclusive view of the body, and certainly a view of the body that includes the active voice of the subject constructing outlandish claims about environments and bodies. Environmental illness, it would seem, is an anomaly, a somatic experience that according to prevailing biomedical theory one should not have.

Anomalies periodically occur in theoretical physics and chemistry with no apparent side effects for the ordinary person (Kuhn 1970). When a human body becomes an anomaly for medicine, however, the effects can be experienced as quite real. An operations clerk writes:

> Upon two occasions I found myself using the emergency room of our local hospital. Upon mentioning my problems with chemicals, I was either ignored or—as one suggested—it was all bunk and proceeded to make fun of my situation and thought I was nuts. Another time I had to have minor surgery in the emergency room and tried to explain to the nurse that the disinfectant she opened up bothered me. Again, I was ignored.

Not all respondents who consulted physicians found them hostile to their nascent theories. In a limited number of cases, people visited doctors who knew something about the controversies over chemicals and the body. A few of them affirmed their patients' work to reclassify their life spaces and manage their symptoms. A housewife writes: "I count myself lucky. The first doctor I went to told me about environmental illness. She said it was something new and it sounded like I might have it."

Her story is unusual, however. Only 9 people among the 121 we interviewed reported visiting physicians who respected their accounts and worked with them to solve the puzzle of EI.[2] In these unusual cases we see how some experts, for whatever reasons, collude with nonexperts, supporting their theories in spite of the resistance of the profession. We will revisit this process in more detail in the final chapter. It is sufficient for the moment to note it and to remember that while it is the exception rather than the rule in our interviews, it can be an important variation in the separation of expert knowledge from expert systems, namely, the separation of an expert from the system.

But whether or not a physician agreed with the initial cause-and-effect reasoning of a person whose body reacts in untoward and debilitating ways to ordinary environments, the point is that this person is making concrete correlations between somatic experiences and putatively benign places and things. "What is real for me," writes a book salesman, "is what I am going through, what I feel like, not what other people tell me I should be feeling, or not feeling." A psychologist with EI writes:

> My degree is in psychology and if I had encountered a client who made claims such as I do, I would have no doubt the person was mentally ill. This illness is so bizarre-appearing and so unbelievable that I have trouble believing it myself! It is only that I experience it myself that allows me to know the truth of it.

A housewife is more direct: "I get dizzy . . . around paint solvents and usually right after I get big, massive headaches. If I get away from the solvents I'm fine. . . . Are you going to tell me it's not the solvents?"

The truth of MCS begins with ordinary people who experience untoward changes in their bodies. If modernity "actively eliminates the idea of the Subject" (Touraine 1995, 27), replacing the unique and personal qualities of the knower by what is objectively known, it might be said that the Subject is returning in the form of a sick body. Knowing that begins with the sensations of the body rekindles an epistemology that is anything but Cartesian, namely, I feel, therefore I think. When bodies resist being the objects of biomedical theory and somatic experiences become a source of objective knowledge, it is not difficult to imagine a fault line in the foundation of modern rationality.

For the chemically reactive, knowledge about their sickness originates with embodied experiences that are typically tracked, classified, and arranged into meaningful clusters. It is a practical epistemology insofar as it joins experiences to practices and is mindful of the results. A former intensive care nurse describes what she would say to a person who wanted to understand this stage in the process of becoming multiply chemically sensitive:

> I would . . . ask the person to take a notebook and for one day write down the chemicals found in every item they eat or drink that day (as listed in the ingredients). Ask them to list every item in their home that is scented, every cleaning product and the chemicals they contain. Chemicals they encounter in stores, gas stations, day cares, etc. What pesticides they used and how often they used them. . . . Then ask them to look up the exposure limits of each and the accumulative effect.

What follows are accounts of how people reorganize their thinking about their bodies and environments by a meticulous, detailed process of assigning somatic responses to ordinary chemical products and routine places. In the language of statistics, associations quickly become correlations as their trial-and-error methods yield a more manageable, but also more circumscribed, world. These several accounts illustrate the obvious fact that truth for the environmentally ill is not being sought outside a deliberately rational practice, though that practice originates, some might say heretically, with human experience.

Reordering and Reclassifying

An attorney describes her first attempts to understand how her body might be responding to her house and to control her exposure:

> Rob and I finally started going through the cabinets. When I would open one and the smell would just overwhelm me, I'd shut it and ask him to get rid of what was in there. . . . We had stuff in the pantry, but that doesn't smell. It was in the bedroom. We have all these hand creams. Like every Christmas somebody would stick some sort of bath oil in your Christmas stocking. . . . So we literally filled up bags of stuff and gave it to my mother and anybody who wanted it. . . . I would open the bathroom cabinet and say, "Well, Rob, I guess some of these towels were washed with fabric softener. I can still smell something. . . . We

got rid of baby powder, shampoo, herbal shampoo, and stuff like that.
. . . Rob got rid of his aftershaves and colognes. . . . There's no more
Comet to clean with. No more Windex or other things like that. . . . I
visited my parents and when I was using their bathroom I had to come
out and say, "Dad, what is in your bathroom? I can't even go in there."
And he said, "Oh, I put some Pine Sol in the toilet. Is that going to
cause you a problem?" I said, "It's driving me bonkers!"

A professional writer, Lynn Lawson (1993), recalls her initial illness
experiences with her house and her day-to-day routines:

First . . . I wanted to clean up my house and lifestyle. . . . My husband
and I had our unvented gas kitchen stove removed and an electric one
installed. We bought air filters that removed chemicals, one for our living room, and one for our bedroom, and one for our car. We started
driving our car with windows closed, the filter going, and the ventilat-
ing system on "recirculate." We try to leave ample space between our
car and other cars' exhaust pipes. My husband reads our daily paper
first, then puts it in a zippered nylon mesh bag and "bakes" it for forty
minutes in our electric dryer vented to the outside, which outgasses
chemicals in paper and ink so that I can read it. . . . I threw out . . .
petroleum-based products. . . . I put away my electric blanket (the
heated wire gives off fumes) and sleep under down, wool, or cotton, as
pure as possible. Essentially it was back to the thirties—to the products
that I remember my mother using. (28)

In addition to becoming aware of local environments as possible
sources of distress, the chemically reactive are likely to use a "first-
this-and-then-that" mode of reasoning to classify somatic changes in
relationship to specific places and things. Some respondents reported
a similar somatic reaction to a wide array of places and things. A legal
secretary and folksinger first lists an array of built environments and
commercial products she correlates with a common symptom pattern.
Among the things that trigger her symptoms are the following:

Petroleum and many of its by-products, herbicides, perfumes, chemical cleaners, brand-new books, all synthetic materials, hospitals,
recently renovated rooms, buildings heated with oil furnaces, places
with air-conditioning. . . .

The first symptoms I notice are usually a growing nausea and an
increasing tremor in my entire body. My head starts to pound and I
begin to feel anxious and jumpy. Then an overwhelming fatigue sets in.
As all these symptoms worsen, my jaw clenches and my shoulders and
neck tense up. After a while I feel like all my insides want to leap out of
my body. . . . I feel extremely uncomfortable and extremely ill.

An art history catalogue editor first lists her symptoms, ranked
according to whether they are chronic or occur occasionally because
of unusual exposures, followed by the places and things that make her
sick:

Symptoms: chronic chemical bronchitis, . . . nasal congestion, digestive
problems, circulation problems in hands and feet, synovitis in one toe
and possible hip joints, extreme sensitivity around root surface of teeth
. . . irritability, impaired memory, recent allergies to dust mites and
mold. The above complaints are unchanging; with prolonged exposure,
I experience extreme fatigue, flulike feeling, pressure on sinuses,
headache, and neuromuscular twitching that interferes with sleep.

The following are some of the places and things that make her sick:

retail stores selling clothing, dry cleaners, beauty salons, new cars, gas
stations, any new building containing emissions from carpeting . . .
vinyl, upholstery, varnish, office copiers, laser printers, Scotch tape,
felt-tip markers, nail polish, hair spray.

Other respondents were more precise in their inventories of environmental triggers and somatic reactions, drawing exact correlations
between one or two offending agents and a specific reaction. A
woman with a bachelor's degree in English who worked as a typesetter for many years recounts her taxonomy:

Gasoline causes anger and pain in the head. . . . Wal-Mart causes gastrointestinal pain and I get very spacey to the point of not even being able to remember my name or do what I went in there for. . . . Fabric softener causes severe back pain so that I'm not even able to walk at times. Living in Louisiana causes back pain and my body cannot hold a chiropractic adjustment . . . because of the massive chemical exposures.

A products designer writes: "When I am exposed to chlorinated solvents . . . I first get stabbing pain behind my eyeballs, my vision blurs, my brain starts to swell. . . . When I am exposed to chlorinated hydrocarbons, however, I have a different set of symptoms."

A former advertising executive is considerably more systematic in her classification scheme. She listed fifty-two separate "Chemicals and Irritants" on the left side of the page and her reactions on the right side. Consider an excerpt from her taxonomy of environmental agents and somatic responses:

Chemicals and Irritants	My Reaction
Polyester	Throat tightens
Clothing dyes	Skin crawls
Newsprint	Body vibrates
Computers	Difficulty concentrating
Magic markers	Nasopharyngeal passages irritated
Synthetics in clothing	Body vibrates
Electricity	Stimulates bladder
Forced-air systems	Pain in neck gland

This same woman goes on to describe how she makes use of her classificatory scheme to sort out the risks she is likely to encounter in accomplishing an ordinary task:

Most people take buying a new watchband for granted. Your old one wears out. You stop in at the local jeweler and you select a new one. The jeweler attaches it to your watch, and you walk out and forget about it. I have learned to take nothing for granted. I ask myself, first, whether this is a day when I can tolerate the environment in the street on the way to the jeweler. If yes, will the air in his store knock me out? Can I tolerate the air long enough to pick out a watchband? . . . Will I react to the chemicals in a leather band? Can I tolerate the plastics and the resins in a man-made watchband?

A former chemical engineer who now makes a living as a substitute teacher has also constructed an elaborate taxonomy of environmental agents and somatic responses:

Auto exhaust	A traveling pain that might first be in my leg, then elbow, etc.
Tertiary amines (ammonias)	Low-level paranoia
Hexane	Fear
Natural gas	Giddiness at low concentrations, grogginess at higher concentrations
Fertilizers	A feeling that the top of my head is coming off
Food additives	Pain in joints

After constructing his taxonomy, he describes a person entering his office as he reads what he has just written: "I am proofreading now, and someone just came in who is wearing perfume, so my thinking ability is reduced as the skin on my back and my lower back is getting tight." Noteworthy in this short aside is its matter-of-fact tone, expressing a "first-this-and-then-that" logic with not so much as a hint of surprise. "Exposure to perfume equals reduced thinking ability" is one of the many ways of correlating bodies and ordinary commercial products that for this person seem rather unremarkable.

A retired file clerk constructs her own taxonomy of unexceptional consumer items and somatic symptoms. Among her many correlations are the following:

Cleaning solvents	Insomnia, memory loss
Most shampoos	Rash on face and muscle pain
Plastic phones	Memory loss, headaches
Answering machines	Burning in neck and shoulders

Gasoline	Severe headaches, insomnia
Bounce fabric softener	Skin discoloring and nausea
Leather shoes	Shortness of breath

A former librarian develops yet another elaborate scheme, a portion of which is reproduced here:

Aspirin, various drugs	Blood pressure surges, burning skin
Scented soaps	Sore throat, severe headache, sometimes congestion, emotions
Plastics	Headache, eyes dry, burning throat, muscle pain/spasms/weakness, thirsty
Street work, asphalt, treated poles	Sore (loose) teeth, temperature rise, blood pressure surges, headache, burning skin, stomach pains, cramps
Toxic plastic phones	Headaches, facial numbness, muscle/joint pains

Not everyone is as precise as the first several excerpts would suggest in relating specific agents with specific somatic responses. Some people construct a more general taxonomy. "Malls," a former seamstress writes, cause "breathing trouble, nausea, dizziness, headaches. fribromyalgia, chronic fatigue syndrome, which is extreme," while "church" causes "severe respiratory distress." A marine transport dispatcher writes, "Houses with vinyl siding are dangerous for me. Even driving by one can cause my eyes to burn. Walking by one I am likely to lose my balance and stumble." He continues, "If I walk into a backyard with a gas grill I often experience memory loss, even if the grill is not working." A retired army colonel developed a rating system to catalogue his varied somatic reactions to environments and his body's capacity to withstand the "insults": "0 to 5 is my 'insult scale.' I figure my body can be only so insulted before it breaks down. . . . Say I've been exposed to two 4s and one 5 in the morning and I am invited to someone's house that evening for dinner. I will usually decline because I will likely get sick if I am exposed to any more insults." Among the twelve 5s on the "insult scale" are "traffic jams," "visits to the Veterans Administration office," "shopping malls," and "filling my car with gas."

The body we encounter in the several narratives on reordering and reclassifying is not the body we encounter in standard biomedical theory and practice. The primary differences are in the perspectives or vantage points from which bodies are considered and in the strategies for classifying them. Consider first the idea of vantage point, or a stance for viewing bodies.

A Return to the Body's Surface

What is essential to know about a body for a person with MCS is what is generally ignored by biomedicine—specifically, its situated relationship with houses, schools, parks, stores, churches, hospitals, shopping malls, and the thousands of commercial products found in these and similar places. The accounts of reclassifying and reordering share the idea that bodies are known in their relationships to environments. A person with MCS examines points of intersection between her body and those places and things it is encountering. She is interested in the surface of her body and its points of contact with material culture.

Biomedicine's gaze, on the other hand, is directed from the physician to the body, and only rarely, if at all, is the relationship between the body and the environment considered in clinical terms. Professional medicine, Foucault reminds us, "project[s] upon the living body a whole network of anatomo-pathological mappings: to draw the dotted outline of the future autopsy. The problem, then, is to bring to the surface that which is layered in depth" (1973, 162). Echoing Foucault, Young writes, "Illness in Western society is viewed from an 'internalizing' perspective. The relevant causes are immediate and localized within the body" (1976, 148; see also Freund and McGuire

1991, 208). Accordingly, the body in biomedicine is defined in the absence of physical, chemical, or social environments.[3]

In reordering and reclassifying their relationship to material culture, the environmentally ill are shifting attention from an interior view of the body to the spaces where bodies and places intersect. For them this is a practical, indeed necessary, shift in perspective. We don't believe the chemically reactive would argue that their version of the body should replace the internal body of biomedicine; clearly, important things occur in the interior of the body. But they would argue for the legitimacy and the complementarity of a version of the body as a porous surface, absorbing the environments it touches. For them, we might say, the truth about the body is that it is many things.

Constructing a practical epistemology is, after all, not a search for universal truth but a deliberate attempt to know something important that is at once empirically and psychologically self-legitimating. "YOU ARE WHAT TOUCHES YOU," announces a flier from the Healthy Environment Info and Referral Service (January 1996), an MCS support group. The announcement continues:

> We aren't only what we eat, we are also what we breathe and touch....
> Our bodies are part of the overall environment exposed to many toxic
> elements. . . . Buildings and monuments everywhere are deteriorating
> from the effects of pollution; our bodies eventually react in the same
> way.

Both a human body and a polished stone shaped into something worthy of remembering can deteriorate at those points where they intersect with dangerous environments. Some observers might find it spurious to compare bodies that appear to get sick when exposed to places and things routinely identified as safe with monuments exposed to acidic rain. The chemically reactive, however, experience their symptoms as legitimate somatic complaints and thus know there is a connection between their disabilities and local environments.

The studied focus of the environmentally ill on the places and things touched and absorbed by the surfaces of their bodies invites comparison with an earlier period when the body's exterior was a source of considerable medical and popular attention. From the 1940s to the 1960s, bodies were imagined as vulnerable to an endless number of microorganisms. Germs were pictured as swarming on the surfaces of material culture—tables, drinking glasses, clothing, and so on—looking for a path into the interior of the body. "Enormous attention," writes anthropologist Emily Martin, "was devoted to cleaning surfaces" that would come in contact with the body, and, in turn, cleaning "surfaces of the body" (1994, 24).[4] The surface of the body was viewed as extremely vulnerable to invasion by germs. "It was the opening left in the body's surfaces—a literal physical breach—that would allow disease to get in" (27).

By the late 1960s, however, biomedicine was focusing its research attention on the immune system, and popular culture was singing the praises of "Your Magic Doctor," or "Our Internal Defender" (Martin 1994, 51). Modern society had discovered a new champion. (It is worth recalling that the first academic department of immunology opened its doors in 1972.) A pathogenic environment could now be rendered innocuous by a robust immune system. Indeed, germs rarely overwhelmed a healthy immune system. Rather, like an invincible army, the immune system seemed to get stronger as it repelled its archenemy. With something inside the body to protect it from disease, we could be less concerned with the body's surface and, for that matter, the cleanliness of the environments it encountered.

The emergence of MCS is once again focusing cultural attention on the surface of the body and surrounding environments, but with a considerably different emphasis than the personal hygiene movement of thirty years ago. Most noticeable is the shift from germs to chemicals as disease-causing agents. Ironically, the very same cleaning products that were advertised to protect against germs, such as Lysol, Borax, and Old English Lemon Oil, to name only a few, are now believed to be the sources of disease. For the chemically reactive, a spotlessly clean environment is probably a genuine health risk.

While both the personal hygiene movement and MCS direct attention to the surface of the body, there are noticeable differences in their respective definitions of risky environments and marked differences in their practical consequences. Dirt, dust, flies, and other germ carriers are unfortunate by-products of entropy and nature, offensive, to be sure, but manageable. The environment of the personal hygiene movement could be washed off the body or neutralized through disinfectants. While countless germs created their own versions of extreme environments, they were nevertheless manageable. The environment of MCS, however, is considerably more insidious, dangerous, and political. Now the very things that protected us from germs make us sick. A chemically reactive person is much less likely to be concerned with dirt than with the commercial products used to remove it. The environment of MCS is literally, to borrow from Giddens (1990), "a manufactured risk." If the personal hygiene movement and its culture of cleanliness helped to create a market for cleaning products that in turn created capital, MCS accuses a capital-producing society of also being a disease-distributing society.

This brief excursus into the pathogenic environment of the personal hygiene movement and its contrasts with the chemically contaminated environment of MCS underscores the importance of medical movements in shaping the way people think about their bodies and environments. And it reminds us of the importance of where in society a movement originates. A professional initiative, the personal hygiene movement configured the authority of medicine with the good offices of federal, state, and local governments, educators, and the prestige presses to construct a persuasive machinery of knowledge and action. The goal of this massive mobilization was to change—control, if you will—such small and seemingly innocuous behaviors as the relationship of the hands to the mouth.

Multiple chemical sensitivity, on the other hand, originates in the perceived failure of the medical profession to explain or acknowledge new and untoward experiences of bodies and environments. Compared with the personal hygiene movement, its goal is considerably more difficult to achieve. The chemically reactive not only must ask others to change routine habits but also must convince powerful institutional others that such changes are warranted—that a new disease is changing the relationship of bodies to places and things typically believed to be safe. Changing the way institutions think, as we will see, requires violating at least a few of their basic assumptions about knowing.

Violating the Generic Body Assumption

A second and related difference between the chemically reactive body and the official body of biomedicine involves the important question of how bodies are to be classified. To be reliable, it is assumed that a medical classification should account for more than one body. Call any poison control center, for example, and a technician will match an aversive agent with a cluster of symptoms. The underlying assumption is that a particular pernicious agent will trigger the same or similar signs and symptoms in all human bodies. When the Centers for Disease Control in Atlanta, Georgia, predicts the particular viruses likely to cause the flu in a coming season and concocts a vaccine, it assumes it is protecting a generic human body. Finally, when a doctor examines a patient, she approaches the body confident that it will be sufficiently like other bodies to classify it as sick or well using standard diagnostic measures. And, if needed, she can prescribe a treatment based on pharmaceuticals that are manufactured as if human bodies are more alike than different.

Perhaps the most essential premise of biomedicine is the coherence and predictability of the body. While it can be short or tall, thin or fat, ugly or attractive, a body is ultimately knowable as a member of a class of bodies. Without the assurance of this premise, biomedicine as a theory and a profession is at risk of defaulting on its promises to classify and control bodies, to render them uniform and knowable.

A striking feature of the narrative accounts found in this chapter, however, is the diverse and seemingly endless number of particular reactions that particular bodies have to particular environments and

the things found in them. Where there should be considerable dupli-
cation of trigger-response patterns among the chemically reactive if
the body is as generic as biomedicine theorizes, there is, rather,
marked diversity. "Just remember," a writer with MCS notes, "we're
all different: what helps one does not always help the other" (Lawson
1993, 318). Hers is an admittedly troublesome counsel to most practicing physicians. How do those with MCS account for this anomaly?
An English professor with severe EI writes:

> My body is like yours and everybody else's insofar as it will change with
> time, mature, grow old, and die. But my body is different from your
> body and your body is different from another's body because each of us
> responds to chemicals in unique ways. I can't assume that what makes
> you sick will make me sick, or sick in the same way.

A former typesetter explains further: "Each exposure is unique as is
each individual (and the total body load at any given time) so you
can't lump them all together and come up with a blanket reaction."
  A concert musician writes:

> My body is a complex chemistry; it shares some things with your body.
> But I have my own genes, my own cells, my own past as healthy and
> sick. How could my body be exactly like yours or somebody else's. . . .
> I think we [medical science] spend too much time looking at how our
> bodies are alike and not enough time looking at how they are different.

"When people say 'Hey, you're nuts. I don't get sick from watching
TV or reading a newspaper,'" a grade school teacher has a ready
response. "I say back, 'Fine, I wish I had your body. Want to switch!?'"
  Read between the lines of stories told by the chemically reactive
and a curious logic appears to be at work. While no two bodies are
likely to respond to the same environmental trigger in the same manner, thus rendering bodies singular and diverse, it is assumed that most
built environments and commercial products can be grouped together
as a class and approached in the "what if" manner we encountered in
chapter 3: "What if they are potential sources of debilitating symp-

toms?" If the body is a discrete entity in the social construction of EI, the extraordinary variability of modern material culture is grouped and classed as extreme, that is, dangerous and to be avoided or approached with caution.

~

Multiple chemical sensitivity becomes a practical epistemology, in part, through the concrete actions of people trying to cope with bizarre and untoward changes in their bodies. The matter-of-fact, almost prosaic, experiences of reclassifying and reordering their local environments are also organizing the minds of the chemically reactive. To paraphrase Geertz (1983, 155), those miseries they think to understand turn out be the minds they find themselves to have.

It is not difficult to see how the practical work of the environmentally ill is also a shift in the social location of theorizing bodies and disease. A more pronounced version of this shift is expressed in the often elaborate pathophysiology stories told by the chemically reactive to account for what specifically troubles them. As we will see, these stories are, among other things, clusters of words that work to persuade others that MCS is a genuine medical disorder. Not surprisingly, many of the words themselves are borrowed from the medical profession.

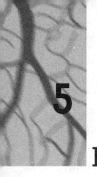

5

Explaining
Strange Bodies

Something so "practical" as a bodily ailment may be a
"symbolic" act on the part of the body which, in this
materialization, dances a corresponding state of mind.

(Burke 1989, 80)

A TURNING POINT for many of the chemically reactive is the
failure of prevailing medical theory and practice to acknowledge their
immediate and tangible somatic experiences. It is worth recalling a
point made briefly in the last chapter. By the time the chemically reactive are seeking the counsel and care of physicians, many of them have
already developed a rudimentary understanding of their troubles.
Matching variable environments and consumer products with variable symptoms, people approaching the medical profession know
something useful about their somatic complaints based on immediate,
tangible experiences.

It is this practical, useful knowledge that is generally unacknowl-
edged by physicians. A physician might listen respectfully to the
accounts of a patient who has catalogued an extensive array of associations between his body and local environments but is not likely to

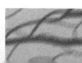

be able to explain these untoward occurrences. In the absence of a professional account of their taxonomic work, the chemically reactive are encouraged to deny the sovereignty of their senses. It would matter little to them to know their situated experiences affirm the modernist assumption that personal experiences must be secondary to professional judgment (Beck 1995; Touraine 1995); to abide by this assumption, however, is to risk their immediate health and well-being.

Between the self of the chemically reactive and the authority of medicine is a recalcitrant, protesting body. Physicians, of course, can attempt to legislate this body, defining it in a manner that allows them to explain it—perhaps telling the patient he suffers from an unusual type of allergy or a neurosis. Or they can reject this body, dedicating themselves to bodies amenable to conventional medical practice. The self in the chemically reactive body, however, cannot, like the peripatetic crab, move out and shop around for a safer home. Unable to emancipate the self from a recalcitrant body, the only other option is to emancipate the self from the authority of the physician. But the act of turning away from a physician will not by itself produce an understanding of why the body is changing.

Like all of us, the environmentally ill are chained to the wheel of meaning, bound by a species need to make sense of their lives. Once associations are made at the immediate moment of the body's response to environments, the self must understand its experiences of a changing body. Perhaps the old saw that "what we don't know can't hurt us" is true some of the time, but for the chemically reactive, knowing can prevent them from being hurt.

The narrative materials in this chapter reveal two interrelated processes: the disenchantment of the chemically reactive with physicians, an often painful process that results in separating biomedical language from the medical profession, and the cognitive work of the environmentally sick to transform their illness experiences into a disease theory using a borrowed medical vernacular.

The Chemically Reactive and the Physician

In this section we will examine why those with MCS are likely to move away from the personification of the medical model, the physician, and toward its most abstract expression: biomedical language. A former nuclear engineer severely disabled by MCS recalls:

> I went to three neurologists, two cardiologists, one rheumatologist, two internists, two hospital clinics for full evaluation including the Mayo Clinic. Also I had been analyzed by two psychologists, one psychiatrist—tested for depression, mental disorders, also medical procedures like MRI, EEG, ultrasound, X-rays repeatedly, and hospitalized three times.

She then summarizes the variety of medical attempts to diagnose her troubles, recalling one physician who admitted her "disease cannot be treated." The rest, however, offered more concrete, if cautious, opinions.

> May be temporal arteritis, may be fibromyalgia, may be conversion reaction disorder, may be scleroderma. . . . The "May be's" kept going on—only a few facts remain the same which all the doctors could not ignore: I am losing my teeth very fast, losing my eyesight, and my eyes are bleeding. . . . And I have severe headaches and hearing loss.

Finally, she makes a plausible argument for the somatic basis of her illness:

> I am not a hysterical person or psycho or faking my symptoms—I was a professional making more than five thousand dollars a month. Now I am living off Social Security disability of nine hundred dollars a month, or 20 percent of my original income. . . . I would have to be stupid or demented to accept that cut in income or status.

For this woman and most of the other chemically reactive people we interviewed, there are few, if any, perceived secondary gains associated with EI.

A graduate student writes regarding her experiences with physicians:

> My overall experience with the medical profession has been varied. I have had the very good fortune to have had several excellent physicians in whom I was able to place my trust. The first, when I lived in New York state, was an internist with many subspecialties, on the faculty of a medical school, and chief of staff of a hospital. Years later, about two and a half years after the crop-dusting incident, when I was still not recovering very well and doctors in this western state did not know what to do with me, I went back to New York to have this internist examine me. After an exhaustive workup (ten days in the hospital) he told me that I had allergies and sensitivities, but he didn't know of an allergist who could adequately treat them in my part of the country, so he put me on Benadryl and sent me home. Three months after returning home I became allergic to the Benadryl and started going downhill rapidly. At one point I was hospitalized (it was during this hospitalization that my first husband left me) and I was told by a local physician at the hospital, "If you don't straighten up, you will die." He never did explain what he meant by "straighten up." I was losing weight rapidly and in a great deal of pain.

In this passage we hear about physicians who are not abandoned by the chemically reactive and do not abandon them, who are resisting the lessons of medical school and the conclusions of medical societies to accept the possibility of a new, incongruous body. When this happens we witness a curious moment: the layperson stepping out of the expert.[1] We will have occasion to say more about maverick experts who step away from their professions and toward citizen movements in the final chapter.

Combining references to philosophy with genuine anger, a former attorney lashes out at the medical profession while acknowledging the importance of physicians who are willing to listen and learn from patients:

Almost invariably, among those who do not specialize in MCS, experiences are very negative—ranging from outright denigration to covert skepticism. Once again, one tries not to see this as personal rejection, but against a sociopolitical-historical background the Cartesian paradigm, science's insistence on visible proof rather than empirical observation, etc. The negativity of the mainstream medical profession, however, is countered by the few dedicated, wonderfully humane doctors we've met who are working in the MCS field—here, they are often persecuted for practicing such heresy, so their stance and support count for much. Once again, an understanding of the pathways of MCS initiation and response provides a good coping mechanism in the face of medical hostility and skepticism. After several abortive tries to find a suitable local physician . . . I found my current local physician, a family practitioner, who, although not terribly knowledgeable about MCS, treats me with respect and as a credible patient, and believes that I have MCS. This physician graciously accepts literature on MCS when I come across it and usually asks me what I can tolerate when I need medication, which does happen occasionally. How refreshing it is to be treated as an intelligent, rational human being with some knowledge of what is good for me and what is not good for me!

A professor of English literature who is on a disability leave recognizes the difficulty physicians face when they encounter the body of the multiply chemically sensitive:

A Social Security psychiatrist diagnosed me as "Schizophrenic, hypochondriacal type." The medical profession has been caring and responsive, doing the best they can with a new and unusual illness or disease that does not fit their models. Their skepticism is understandable—for example, when I tell my urologist my prostate inflammation is caused by breathing wood smoke in the winter, he thinks he's speaking with a fool, because there is *no* training at med school to suggest inflammation comes from environmental exposure.

A legal secretary is less sympathetic with her doctors. She describes herself as:

> very angry about the fact that several doctors I have seen failed to even question that my illness could have been something other than bronchitis, sinusitis, or asthma. Over a period of nine years I saw the same clinic of allergists (three doctors) and not one of them ever suggested anything other than allergy injections, nasal and bronchial inhalers, cortisone, and antibiotics in response to my continued deterioration of health. Even after I explained my extreme reactions to perfume, no one ever suggested that it might be MCS/EI, including the pulmonary specialist and ENT.

Evident in her story and those recounted earlier is the routine failure of physicians to normalize their patients' somatic distress. Whether it is called temporal arteritis, fibromyalgia, allergy, a neurotic-somatizing disorder, or one of hundreds of other standard medical diagnoses, from the vantage point of the chemically reactive, the definition does not match the misery, nor obviously does it cure it.

A professional writer offers a somewhat unflattering explanation for why physicians persist in trying to fit MCS into something they know rather than expand what they are prepared to know:

> I have found that most physicians lack intellectual curiosity, and when faced with a patient who doesn't conveniently fit into their medical mold, they prefer to discard the patient into their medical wastebasket, rather than revise their medical paradigm. With only a very few, notable exceptions, conventional medicine has been a huge disappointment for me. Most of these practitioners have an ego that gets in the way of listening to the patient and a strong, strident bias against anecdotal evidence.

An orchestra conductor summarizes how many people with MCS feel about the medical profession:

> My experiences with the medical profession have been appalling—even horrifying. These people are generally callous, abusive, self-important,

insecure persons who care far more about their cultish allegiance to 1940s medical texts, and the reputation they believe they will maintain thereby, than to human life or any oath to protect it. Most are, at best, smugly complacent.

Finally, consider the words of a man with severe MCS and no medical insurance:

> As I was too poor, with no medical insurance, to go to many doctors, I haven't had to deal with them. The two doctors I did see in six years told me that they didn't know how to treat me. I went to the emergency room at a Little Rock, Arkansas, hospital once after passing out from a chemical overload. The attending physician thought I was "crazy"; I thought him an "old fool."

Worlds collide in these accounts. The physical, painful, mysterious body of the chemically reactive crashes against the orthodox knowledge and practice of a powerful profession. Unable to take a proper measure of this body, to fit it into what physicians know about bodies, it becomes an unwelcome anomaly. What is a concrete and disabling disorder for the chemically reactive is, simply, medically impossible for the physician; thus the patient is "crazy" and the doctor a "fool." A woman with severe EI concludes her account of experiences with the medical profession with the following counsel: "I formulated the only two rules for MCS that always hold true in all circumstances: 1. Nobody knows anything. 2. Nothing makes sense."

Between the lines of the several accounts just presented are two contradictory orders of knowledge: a personal and visceral way of knowing and an authoritative claim that one cannot talk reasonably in these terms. "The biomedical model," writes a professor of medicine and psychiatry, "embraces . . . reductionism, the philosophic view that complex phenomena are ultimately derived from a single primary principle." In this case the nonexperiential, purely "physicalistic . . . language of chemistry and physics will ultimately suffice to explain biological phenomena" (Engle 1977, 90).

A key to understanding modernity is the authority of expertise to disempower the senses (Beck 1995; Touraine 1995). From physics, to biology, to sociology, we are taught that the world is not what it appears to be; we should not trust what we know, or feel, or see. A physician warns his medical colleagues who might be tempted toward acknowledging the validity of a patient's personal story about his body:

> To allow more than objects to enter our experience [as doctors]—*really* enter—would entail a painful reassessment of who we are. It would mandate a redefinition of our relationship to the world, a renunciation of the ordinary subject-object way we habitually define ourselves. (Dossey 1984, 5)

The promise of modernity captured in this physician's warning to his colleagues is easily discerned: surrender the sovereignty of your senses to the authority of administrative expertise, and in return you will enjoy the benefits of legitimate and reliable knowledge about your body, your self, and the world you inhabit.

A woman writes as if she is challenging the legitimacy of this promise:

> I have to be aware of my environment, and my body's reaction to it, subjective or objective. (By the way, technically, the environment includes that which we take internally, such as artificial sweeteners, and drugs—anything which is non-self.) This is a part of trusting myself. To ignore this is to risk serious illness for a long time, even death. I try not to be paranoid and don't think that I usually am paranoid. I only wish I had learned to pay attention to the "wisdom of the body" a lot sooner.

On the body as a source of reliable knowledge, consider the thoughtful, if somewhat prickly, observations of a retired grade school teacher:

> I think the diagnosis of MCS is correct because I obviously do not have *Candida* anymore according to a stool analysis done last year, I am not chronically fatigued anymore, and, with proper testing in an environ-

mental unit, I am sure many of my reactions could be replicated in a single-blind manner the same way they are repeated when I get exposed to whatever is causing them. I trust my body, not my MD. . . . I think my common sense has always been there although the medical profession and circumstances did their best to obliterate it. I feel more strongly about it now than at any other time in my life. Now, it's here to stay.

The credibility of modern medicine, for this woman at least, is a matter of institutional commitments and not of explanatory coherence. Refractory bodies cannot be ignored. They intrude into consciousness and demand to be explained. It is an unusual person who can adapt to a disabled body in the absence of a reasonable account of how and why she became sick. The chemically reactive people we interviewed are anything but unusual, at least on this one measure. Without the benefit of a standard medical diagnosis, they have fashioned their own medical realities, borrowing liberally from the grammar of biomedicine. Forced to become students of their recalcitrant bodies, they continue to monitor their somatic reactions and search relevant literatures, particularly the research literature on MCS.

Constructing a Practical Epistemology

A woman who has lived with the illness for over twenty years recalls her first efforts to know what was happening to her body: "I started studying, reading everything I could get my hands on. I have quite an extensive library but there's so much coming out that I'm getting behind. I have books, newsletters, tapes."

"After no help from a poorly trained MD," writes one man, "I started reading and making phone calls. . . . you just have to take control of your medical needs." A bookkeeper notes, "I read everything I can find and doctor myself." A woman with MCS encourages fellow sufferers to "be your own private detective agency. Look for clues everywhere. . . . You can never know too much about this stuff" (Lawson 1993, 318). Another woman acknowledges the relationship of knowledge to personal empowerment: "I avidly go after any information I can find on MCS and related issues. I've become a source others recommend for information; and a fine investigative journalist I know says I ought to be an investigative journalist."

A young woman with severe MCS describes the process by which she has created her own library:

> I first learned about MCS by reading a letter to an editor in my local newspaper (at the time I was living in Baton Rouge, Louisiana). It was the first time that I had ever read anything that so closely described my personal experience. It was virtually biographical! I contacted the organization that had sponsored the letter (HEAL of Louisiana). . . . It was Diane who opened her heart and her personal library to me. I try to return this gift, every day, when I receive calls from "novice" EIs. I remember starting a single file folder headed "EI/MCS." Now I have two rooms (home offices) full of file cabinets and bookshelves. My husband teases that we will soon have to build an addition to our house, to warehouse all my books, files, videos, etc.

In a more restrained admission of the importance of literature on making sense of somatic experiences, one man writes:

> Well, I read about MCS in newspaper articles and books as I tried to figure out why I was ill. I read about multiple chemical sensitivities in relationship to cleaning up one's environment and realized the symptoms were the same as those for chronic fatigue syndrome. Then I began to notice how symptoms intensified after driving in car fumes, being exposed to a new building.

For this man, literature and secondary associations became a substitute for physicians' counsel.

> I first learned about MCS from an article given to me by a previous roommate. After that, I contacted the Environmental Health Network and did research on my own to learn more about the illness. I then determined that I was chemically sensitive even though I had not been diagnosed at that time by a physician because I lacked insurance.

A middle-age man links his natural curiosity to his search to find out about his disease, justifying his work by acknowledging that, like other living creatures, he too can be poisoned:

> I don't remember how I first learned about MCS. I am a very curious
> person, always investigating and learning. My first indication was from
> the doctor who identified the phenol poisoning. That gave me a starting
> point and then magazines like Sierra Club, Greenpeace, and CMC pub-
> lications. After all, I am an animal, too, and can be hurt just like other
> fauna.

A woman explains why knowledge is a practical necessity: "I learn all I can because I intend to *be well.*" Echoing her intent to learn, another chemically reactive person writes, "I've become a student of my body and of this illness. I read extensively in order to understand MCS and how best to treat it." "Once you find the cause," one man writes, simply, "you have the cure." His optimism, however, is not shared by everyone. A beautician notes, "The last two years I have read everything I can find about MCS to cope with this problem. . . . What is a puzzle to me is I have tried to build my system up to over-come this problem and it just doesn't work." Becoming students of their bodies' disorders did not in fact result in cures for any of the respondents, but each recognized the importance of learning to suc-cessfully cope with their troubles. A retired real estate manager acknowledges the importance of learning about bodies and environ-ments to adapting: "I have done a lot of research on my own and have found some things that help me deal with this horrible illness."

While other respondents wrote longer accounts than those pre-sented here and some wrote shorter ones, the pattern of ordinary peo-ple engaged in constructing a way of knowing that is adequate to comprehend the untoward changes in their bodies is evident in all of the interviews. In the talk of the chemically reactive we see the work involved in fashioning a knowledge about bodies in the absence of medical recognition that real, somatic problems exist.

A common theme in these narratives is the sense of responsibility the chemically reactive assume for knowing the body and its relationship to environments. Their survival is directly linked to the knowledge they produce through systematic observation of their bodies, accompanied by medical and technical reports and conversations with others. To survive MCS, they believe they must know more than the medical professions and most physicians about somatic responses to specific environments. If the boundary between expert and layperson is wearing thin, it is because ordinary people are increasingly forced to theorize their mundane miseries, often in the face of hostile or doubting experts. As we will see in the final chapter, knowing more than the expert whose job it is to know is an increasingly common survival strategy in a society fashioned by a growing number of seemingly unmanageable risks.

Accounting for how and why the chemically reactive learn, however, is only one part of the story. A second, and critical, part is *what* they learn. Under considerable pressure to supply precise understandings of their refractory bodies, the chemically reactive must satisfy not only themselves but others of the legitimacy of their disorder.

Explaining Bodies and Environments

The following passages narrate the work of people who need to conceptualize their troubled bodies. Here abstractions meet somatic complaints, and together they constitute a new, practical epistemology: a sensible, local, and instrumental way of knowing bodies and environments. The clusters of words used by the chemically reactive to explain their bodies are, more often than not, borrowed liberally from the vernacular of biomedicine. A former computer programmer believes he "must sound like a doctor to convince other people and myself, I guess, that all this crap I go through is real, natural, not just mental."

Fashioning biomedical accounts of the etiology and pathophysiology of their disorders allows the chemically reactive to know what they are experiencing and in turn informs their experiences of the disorder. In their work to understand their misery, the chemically reactive are blurring the conventional boundaries between illness and disease, a topic we will return to at the end of this chapter. For the moment, however, it is enough to comment on some properties of the narratives themselves.

First, note the diversity of biomedical accounts of MCS. Indeed, some people ascribe to an entirely different name for the disorder. The lack of a common, agreed upon nomenclature for EI adds considerably to the deliberative work of determining just what is wrong and why. Multiple chemical sensitivity remains a local, individual, or, at most, a small-group problem. While resources are available at regional and national levels in the form of newsletters, tapes, books, and so on, there is little common ground for reaching a shared definition of the disorder. At this point in its development, an explanation of MCS is truly a local knowledge. In spite of their parochial character, however, most definitions do share a common feature.

Regardless of the variable clusters of words chosen by those with MCS to represent their sick bodies, the theories of chemical reactivity constructed in these accounts almost invariably link the body to the external environment. For the environmentally ill, environments can no longer be understood as outside the body. Healing a sick body begins with a working knowledge of the physical and chemical settings to which it is inextricably linked. Most of us conceive of a boundary between our bodies and external environments. We are accustomed to thinking along such lines as "This is where I stop and nature, wilderness, the neighborhood, and so on begins." For the chemically reactive, however, knowing a body is inseparable from knowing the chemistry immediately surrounding it. The following five narratives illustrate both the diversity of lay disease theories and the often technical language used to explain them.

An inventor and sales representative explains his disorder in the highly stylized language of immune system medicine. Realizing he might be confusing a sociologist, he moves from a more difficult to an easier explanation of his troubles:

I personally do not like the term MCS or EI or chemical hypersensitivity. I like the term toxic response symptom. I like an inappropriate
inflammatory affected lymphocyte profile, but we must communicate.
The easiest description is that the chemicals have developed a binding
site on proteins that arouse the immune system to produce too many
helper cells that proliferate throughout the body and interfere with my
body's ability to expel the unwanted chemicals. I lack adequate detox
enzymes to protect me from these toxic chemicals so they cause damage
to cells and autoimmune system.

A graduate student believes her troubles are caused by problems
with her vascular system. "Countless exposures to supposedly safe
chemicals over twenty-eight years are causing my blood vessels to
become weakened and inflamed. Parts of my body are no longer getting an adequate supply of blood. I believe this is the source of my
chronic pain."

A massage therapist directs attention to the importance of the limbic system in explaining MCS:

In my opinion, the theory with the most merit . . . in explaining the
symptoms, according to the results of research, is that the limbic system
of the brain has been damaged by chemical exposure. The limbic system,
also known as the "animal brain," controls basic bodily processes, reg-
ulates both the endocrine and the immune systems, contains the "search
function" for our memories, and influences our emotions. Inhaled chemicals are known to migrate directly to the brain via the olfactory (smell)
nerves. The sensitized limbic system reacts abnormally to these exposures. This has been documented through sophisticated technology such
as the SPECT scan. This abnormal brain response then impacts the rest
of the body, resulting in the many diverse symptoms of MCS.

A man who lives on a boat off the Maryland shore narrates his version of MCS:

I don't have the ability to be exposed to certain families of toxic chemicals. . . . the toxic chemicals accumulate and store in my fatty tissue.

This then activates my immune system and causes autoimmunity and an inappropriate inflammatory process that then lacks the immune component that turns off the activation. Any organ or tissue can be the target of immune attack. After enough attacks, the organ or tissue dies.

A retired navy officer explains MCS as resulting from "a deficiency in the enzymes in my body that are supposed to neutralize toxic chemical substances that I encounter in my day-to-day activities. . . . Enzymes are proteins that work to clean up the body. Mine are not working."

In each of these accounts, the source of MCS is located outside the body—for example, in "certain families of toxic chemicals." Theorizing relationships between modern material culture and sick bodies often occurs in tandem with a language of moral accountability. Fusing technical and medical talk with the rhetoric of social or environmental justice ensures that EI, however it is defined, is both a disease theory and a form of social criticism. In this way MCS is not only a collective representation of problems with bodies and environments; it is also a representation of imperfections in the body politic.

A middle-aged man who works as a substitute teacher and sells automobile insurance explains his disorder using a mix of cellular, evolutionary, and moral appeals:

MCS is a central nervous system response to dangers that we are not consciously aware of. At some point, the central nervous system senses a chemical danger that could in high enough doses cause an injury or disease. . . . Since the first single-cell organism, organisms have been responding to low concentrations of chemicals. . . . Humans have a more complex reaction to poisons than many other species. . . . We delegate portions of our populations to work with chemicals so others can have leisure. We tolerate poisons to make our homes or selves look better. . . . In an effort to save the organism, the sensing organ ups the volume of its output. The nose or skin . . . senses chemical concentrations and tries to say to the body, "Get out of here. You are in danger." If the body doesn't listen, the sending sensory nerve cells up their output volume until the body can hear.

An unemployed legal secretary and office manager understands her disorder as involving immune, limbic, and olfactory systems. She finds it particularly difficult to live with because it is "invisible" to others and renders the body unpredictable.

> Chemical sensitivity is an illness where a person has severe reactions to low levels of chemicals which are used in almost everything we use in our lives, to prescription drugs, and to foods. A person becomes chemically sensitive by either a long-term overexposure to low levels of chemicals, including, but not limited to, new carpets and other building materials, chemical spills, pesticides, etc. Manifestations of MCS may include body swelling, rashes, violent convulsive coughing, chronic fatigue, severe muscle aching, problems focusing eyes, short-term memory loss and inability to concentrate, stomach and other organ problems, and numerous other symptoms. Usually a person with MCS manifests many of these symptoms all at once and they become very depressed. Their bodies have become so toxic that their immune systems have been damaged to the point that they are literally unable to tolerate even traces of chemicals in products they have used all their lives and which others use with no reaction. Chemicals undetectable by the olfactory senses cause them to experience acute symptoms which frequently leave them too weak to function. MCS patients have different levels of damage. Some require oxygen to go outside. Some must wear masks at all times because they can't take the chance of being exposed to anything that will cause them to react. Many cannot even tolerate their own living environment. Sometimes, MCS patients' immune systems are so weakened that they must use a wheelchair or walker to get around. Many chemically sensitive individuals look perfectly normal, not sick at all. MCS is an invisible disability, and because of that many people don't believe it exists. This lack of belief by others and the fact that MCS patients cannot trust their bodies any more not to betray them in public are very difficult to deal with.

A retired professional woman starts her account by building a technical case for her troubles, but she ends on a note of earnest appeal:

The condition is basically one of immune system dysfunction (sometimes called autoimmune disease), but it is not AIDS. The body becomes hypersensitive to a multitude of external and even internal triggers (such as mold, dust, pollen, gases, chemical fumes, even its own hormones). This hypersensitivity produces a host of severe symptoms in a variety of organ systems of the body including debilitating fatigue and muscle weakness, migraine headaches, depression, edema, skin rashes, and inability to concentrate. The body may even attack its own cells and tissues. It is a frustrating and sometimes depressing illness, and while I try to remain optimistic and upbeat, I could use your help, support, encouragement, and understanding.

A professional writer explains MCS as a "chemical injury":

Only a small percentage of the population exhibit what we've come to accept as "allergies." This is really an altered state of reactivity to some benign environmental substance (e.g., pollen). MCS is a diagnosis that refers to "chemical injury" on exposure to substances that have a potential for harm to everyone, when presented in a large enough dose. For example, there is *no safe* level of exposure for formaldehyde. Pesticides contain known neurotoxic agents. My heightened reactivity is in response not to pollens but to synthetic chemicals that are recognized within the scientific community as requiring "threshold limit values" and "permissible exposure limits." Their "risk assessments," however, protect only a portion of society. They haven't safeguarded my health.

A disabled orchestra conductor explains her disorder as if she is talking to others, suggesting the importance of a disease theory in constructing a legitimate social identity:

I think MCS is the correct diagnosis, given the current usage of the term; but I don't believe "MCS" is a diagnosis at all, in that it is merely descriptive. I understand that "MCS" was coined by an MD who was antagonistic to the recognition of the disease. My objection is that it says nothing of the mechanism, or what it is. I prefer "RUDS (reactive upper airways disease) with toxic encephalopathy." To a nonscientific friend, I will simply say I'm "chemically sensitive" or "chemically reactive." At times, with certain people, I have no objection to their understanding that I am "allergic to chemicals." In the common usage of "allergy," this is not terribly inaccurate. I am, however, very quick to correct mistaken MDs, and those who try to trap me: "Oh, so you feel you're allergic to chemicals?" they say with that condescending tone. I snap back, "Not IgE," and go on to present a plausible biomedical model, which invariably causes their eyes to glaze over.

As the preceding narrative suggests, distinguishing MCS from allergies is important to many people who are theorizing their bodies' intolerance to chemicals and environments. Biomedical accounts of normal allergies locate the source of the disorder in the body, specifically in hypersensitive IgE antibodies that mistake ordinary environmental agents, pollen, dust, and so on, as toxic. For the chemically reactive, however, the problem does not originate in their bodies but in chemically saturated environments. The distinction is important for many reasons, not the least of which is its mandate to expand the medical gaze beyond the body to include houses, stores, streets, parks, offices, and libraries, among hundreds of other places, as possible sources of disease.

Note how language is used in the following accounts to distinguish MCS from allergies. A retired computer program analyst explains:

> The term allergy generally refers to a genetic disorder that involves acute . . . reactions mediated by an antibody called immunoglobulin E. I don't have this. My problem is an acquired one that comes from toxic overexposure and produces delayed reactions which can come in response to very tiny amounts of airborne contaminants, . . . food additives, and some foods (the list of which is always changing).

A phone consultant describes environments and chemicals filling bodies, an etiology story far different from that of IgE-mediated allergies.

MCS is an accurate diagnosis of my illness because I react to all chemical substances in a negative way. It's not an allergy. As I go through my daily routine I am exposed to various chemicals. Once I reach my total body load, I have a reaction. Some days it may take longer depending on exposures and this confuses people, as they may see that I have briefly visited a mall. However, my symptoms can be turned on and off like a light switch. Expose me to a chemical, and I will have a reaction. Spray the room with bug spray and when I enter my vision will dim or I will become aggressive or feel strange, without even knowing it has been sprayed. The reaction depends on what I have been exposed to prior to that exposure. Not all reactions are the same and this confuses people. Take me away from all man-made materials and chemicals, including our outside environment, and I will feel mostly normal as long as I don't read or clean the house or do anything that might result in a reaction. However, prolonged exposure to my own home causes fatigue and brain fog. I must change environments at least twice a day to detox.

A farmer contextualizes MCS by locating its origin outside the body, accuses an allergist of causing a toxic reaction, and suggests the disorder is reaching pandemic proportions.

I think MCS is an accurate diagnosis because my illness was precipitated by Agent Orange poisoning and I react to many chemicals, in addition to natural allergens, and my reactions rarely produce antibodies but rather symptoms of poisoning. For example, my digestive tract reacts more like I have eaten arsenic than a common allergen like a banana. My respiratory tract acts like (especially burning) I have inhaled a poison like sulphur rather than a common allergen like pollen. I became allergic to molds only after the allergist poisoned me with phenol in conjunction with a mold allergen. And since when is it normal—or at least natural—for everybody to have allergies? Fifty percent of the population of Chico (or more now) have "allergies." This may be "normal" but it is not natural. It is artificially induced ill health in an entire population surrounded by farm country and sprayed public lands. I also don't think MCS is an adequate term. I think something like multiple artificially induced sensitivities (MAIS) would be more appropriate. The only "allergies" I had all my life before the Agent Orange poisoning were to milk and poison oak. Now hundreds of substances disable me with MCS while giving other people less obvious reactions—cancer, leukemia, CFIDS, MS, Parkinson's, etc. Poisoning is epidemic!

A retired accountant uses allergy as a metaphor to explain how MCS is different:

Multiple chemical sensitivity is somewhat akin to an allergy, in that we get sick from things that don't affect other people. But, in many ways it's far more serious than getting hay fever from the cat or from pollen. People with MCS react to things that are all around them, everywhere they go: things like plastics and carpets and perfumes. And their reactions can be far more serious than sneezes and spots. Some people might suffer blinding headaches or become paralyzed. Others might become hyperactive or violent. And others might be unable to remember things, or to concentrate enough to learn at school, or to function as members of society. It's all very individual: everyone has different reactions, which may affect any part of the body, and reacts to different things. This is what makes it so hard for the average doctor to diagnose or understand—and for the unaffected person to accept. This often makes it difficult for the patient, who may find it hard to cope with rejection and disbelief, on top of his illness. Some people are so sensitive, to so many things, that they are forced to live in virtual isolation. While such a situation may seem incredible to the unaffected person, there are many people—all over the Western world—in this situation.

One observation seems rather obvious from these accounts: EI is not a single, coherent practical epistemology. It should perhaps be thought of as a discrete, highly personal resource for talking about bodies, environments, and society. Separating languages of expertise from expert systems and locating them in situated, personal lives ensures that the chemically reactive are, to paraphrase Geertz (1983, 10), constructing texts ostensibly medical out of local, biographical experiences. Each of the narratives recounted here bears characteristic marks of a unique self. Environmental illness is less a collective representation of bodies and environments and more an invitation to think through the immediate, tangible, and particular relationships between a self, its body, and its chemical surroundings. Its particular rather than universal mode of reasoning makes it infinitely adaptable to the needs of discrete persons and their sick bodies, though it violates a condition of rational knowledge that it must be generalizable.

Interpreting Theories

What are we to make of these highly variable, often moral, accounts of the etiology and pathophysiology of MCS, EI, or one of their corollary terms? The question can be approached from several vantage points. A good place to begin is with the problem of knowledge and the environmentally ill body itself.

A sick body insists on being understood. It is almost as if the disorder of a body requires the order of a text. As in this case, a body experienced as chemically reactive encourages a pattern of thought about environments, immune systems, limbic systems, central nervous systems, and so on.[2] Human sickness reminds us of a somewhat messy proposition, namely, the question of how we know bodies cannot be separated from the question of how bodies know. It is worth a brief foray into the more well-known strategies for addressing the idea that bodies are both objects and subjects, a topic several of our respondents addressed in one way or another.

Foucault (1977) addresses the dual properties of the body by ignoring its agentic possibilities. His body is simply the product of language, a discursive object of control and surveillance. For anthropologist Margaret Lock (1993), the body is more than a state-sponsored language; it is also "an active forum for the expression of dissent and loss" (141). For the teenager who pierces his lips and nose with rings, the body is a physical location for symbolizing separation from authority and attachment to others who are perhaps also piercing their bodies. The idea of the body as an expression of belonging and dissent is a corrective to Foucault's exclusively normative body, but both approaches examine a body as an object acted upon by the state or the self. How would the chemically reactive respond to Foucault's and Lock's notions of the body as a social construct, an expression of order and dissent?

A retired Navy officer is troubled by "psychiatrists and psychologists who make their living telling us it's all in our heads. I told a shrink, 'my head listens to my body.' He smiled and continued to ask me questions about my anger." Examine a number of comments culled from the interviews that strike a similar note: "I believe what I experience"; "I know what I feel"; "If I doubt my body I doubt my mind"; and "Throughout the day I listen to what my body is telling me. If I don't I can find myself in some real pickles."

Finally, consider these comments made by a primary school teacher: "I trust my body. It's the only thing that has been predictable throughout this craziness. . . . If I listen to a doctor, many of them anyway, I probably stay sick or get sicker. But if I listen to my body it tells me what to do to survive."

Contrary to Foucault and others who would see bodies as little more than clusters of authoritative words or physical expressions of dissent, the chemically reactive believe their bodies know things. These quotes express an assumption that bodies possess extradiscursive properties that are important, in some instances, for survival. For those with MCS, perceiving and knowing are not exclusively activities of the self or the state but are shaped in part by the body and its relationships to environments. For them, the body participates in the structure of their imagination; as it changes, becoming less tolerant of modern commodity culture, it encourages them to rethink what they know about their physical selves and the environments surrounding them.

If visceral knowledge is not reducible to culture, however, it is only through culture that such knowledge is represented. And it should come as no surprise to learn that the organization of modern commodity culture discourages the representation of body knowledge (Martin 1990; Sheets-Johnstone 1992). We are more apt to attend to the messages of popular culture regarding our bodies than to our bodies themselves. Male and female fashion models, nutritionists, pharmacological researchers, physicians, and weight and fitness experts are among the many voices that speak for bodies. For one commentator, "The living sense of ourselves vanishes in the din of popular body noise" (Sheets-Johnstone 1992, 3). The body as commodity overshadows the body as a source of prediscursive wisdom. If the Cartesian revolution reduced appreciably the voice of the body as a source of knowledge, its successful appropriation by market forces rendered it nearly mute.

The environmentally ill body, however, is fashioned, for all practical purposes, without the benefit of institutional representation—indeed, in opposition to it. In a culture where visceral knowledge is expropriated and replaced by languages of advertisers and physicians who know best, crediting the body with its own authoritative voice is likely to be accomplished in a language of opposition and difference. Throughout chapters 3 and 4 we encountered languages of opposition created by the chemically reactive to give voices to their troubled bodies.

The environmentally ill body appears to encourage imaginative work expressed in a language of biomedicine that is opposed both to the medical profession and to the built and modified environments of modern commodity culture. Specifically, EI is a lingual resource for constructing the unsettling idea that commodity culture itself is, in fact, sick—contagiously so. In this fashion MCS becomes clusters of words for representing bodies protesting their troubled relationships with much of the material of modernity.

There is in fact one area where these diverse narratives converge: etiology. A dizzying number of pathophysiological possibilities are embedded in these accounts. Advocates for central nervous, limbic, or immune system disorders vie with advocates for upper airway obstructions, brain inflammation, and the somewhat general chemical injury, among other accounts of what is sick. This diversity of disease pathway stories, however, is not matched by a diversity of disease origin stories. While there are some biographical differences in the specifics of causality (acute versus chronic, for example), all accounts of EI—including those found in chapter 3—locate its origins in pathogenic or sick environments. As theories of the sources of sick bodies, etiologies are inevitably moral and political accounts. While causality is never really independent of casuistry, the rhetoric of biomedicine would have us believe the origin of disease is almost invariably in an amoral, natural body.

Biomedical language routinely transforms somatic complaints into a powerful rhetoric of naturalism that locates sources and solutions in the chemistry and physiology of the body (Martin 1987; Kozak 1994). Physicians and medical researchers routinely use biomedical language to depoliticize diseases by locating their origins in the body (Sontag 1989; Lock 1993). For their part, physicians do not intentionally obscure the social, political, or environmental origins of disease. Rather, they routinely treat bodily symptoms, seeking, as their licenses proscribe, to treat the sick body. The net result of this approach, however, is the idea of the body as the origin and site of disease. From this vantage point, the body is indifferent to moral appeal; it is neither good nor bad, just sick. One can blame the person for getting sick, of course, but that is beside the point in the clinical encounter, where the emphasis is on a cure.

In spite of the fact that modern medicine denies the value of certain kinds of relationships—putatively benign environments and disease, for example—those relationships remain linguistically available to individuals as a basis for generating an alternative way of understanding what makes bodies sick. The practical necessarily becomes political as the chemically reactive argue for the origin of disease outside of their bodies, specifically in putatively benign built and modified environments. Their narrative accounts contain an alternative strategy for the origin, development, and deployment of medical knowledge.

Finally, with a few exceptions, the patterns of thinking recounted in the narratives presented in this chapter include an extrarational, often emotional, moral appeal. Two orders of persuasion—the technical and the moral—are joined here into one account (see Chapter 2). While a moral appeal typically enjoys more credibility than one grounded in an alleged physical reality, combining the two expands considerably the number of venues a person can hope to influence (Epstein 1991, 1995). Perhaps the practical epistemology of EI heralds a new strategy for citizen action.

Most social movements share a populist appeal to rights and entitlements based upon the idea of citizenship (Waltzer 1991; Seligman 1992). A rhetoric of moral entreaty fashions appeals to freedom of speech, thought, and faith, the right to own property, the right to economic welfare, the right to clean environments, and so on. In social movements, moral understandings of right and wrong, good and bad, proper and improper are created, affirmed, and changed (Gusfield 1963).

Like their counterparts in the feminist, labor, and civil rights movements, those in the environmental movement typically appeal to issues of justice and rights to make their claims. At the end of the nineteenth century and the beginning of the twentieth century, for example, people organized in response to a perceived need to protect and conserve species and habitats (Schnaiberg 1980; Nash 1989). Their moral appeal was based on accepting a transition from liberalism's natural rights philosophy to a "rights of nature" ethic (Nash 1989, 7). More recently, appeals to environmental justice and the more provocative charge of environmental racism direct attention to unequal distributions of risks (Szasz 1994).

The environmentally ill, however, are organizing around more than a populist appeal to moral or ethical rights. Specifically, people who believe they are made sick by the production, use, and disposal of modern material culture are fusing a moral appeal for safe environments with a popular appropriation of biomedical knowledge to make a particularly persuasive claim on institutions to change or modify their behaviors and policies. We find this development interesting for its representation of the complex exchange between citizens, expert knowledge, and expert systems in the waning years of the twentieth century.

If Locke could write in the seventeenth century that the "rights of man" would be assured by joining the ordinary person to "instrumental rationality," by the nineteenth century ordinary people were effectively separated from technical ways of knowing the world. From the early twentieth century to the present, appeals to human rights were increasingly dissociated from rationality and its instruments (Touraine 1995). Expert knowledge was the province of the professions, licensed and protected by the state (Giddens 1990).

Expert systems emerged, mysterious and complicated, almost magical, artfully manipulating weights and measures, microscopes, slide rules, tests of all sorts—in short, the instruments of rational knowledge. Social movements relied on ethical and moral, not scientific, appeals to lobby for change. If an expert opinion was needed, the best a person or group could do was to hire an expert to represent their interests. Sociologists wrote about "symbolic politics" (Gusfield 1963, 180) and "rhetorics of transcendence" (Stewart, Smith, and Denton 1984, 121). Ordinary citizens could certainly appeal to scientific ways of knowing to assist them in constructing a rhetorical message, but they were not themselves claiming to know something new and legitimate based on their use of scientific knowledge. Separating citizens from instrumental rationality ensured that modernity would succeed, as Alain Touraine (1995) writes, in separating the "world of nature, which is governed by the laws discovered and used by rational thought, and the world of the Subject" (57).

But nature and the Subject cannot avoid one another in the embodied narrative of EI. Environmental illness is a story constructed by nonexperts about human bodies in somatic dissent against a material world saturated with commodities promising to make life easier and healthier, and the body itself more attractive. It is a survival story and thus ultimately a moral story, one told in a language of instrumental and rational action.

A reasonable and final question to ask of these narratives is whether they are true. A practical epistemology may or may not meet medical or scientific criteria of truth; its standard of validity is more immediately sensible and can be summed up in the question Does it work? or Is it useful? A practical epistemology reclaims ordinary experience as a pathway to knowledge. Based on immediate, tangible, and sensory evidence of cause and effect between bodies and environments, EI reconciles the self and the body. It restores a sense of order between the cognitive, emotional, and somatic parts of a person. In short, while it is not a cure, the story of EI may help a person to heal. "I sometimes wonder if MCS is real," a mother and housewife writes, "I mean, a lot of people think it isn't. But then I think, 'Well, are you better now than you were when you didn't know what was wrong?'... If I'm a kook, okay, at least I feel better."

"When I read about environmental illness," recalls a retired engineer, a light went on in my head and I said, 'Ha-ha, I'm not crazy.' Knowing what was wrong with me has been important. I can explain myself now." A former advertising executive is more to the point: "MCS is not a cure, it is a way to stay alive and not just physically alive. I mean psychologically alive."

Staying "physically" and "psychologically alive" through telling stories about environments and bodies framed in the borrowed language of biomedicine is a pragmatic response to the question, Yes, but are these stories true? If a new body is emerging in society, however, it will need to satisfy more than the chemically reactive themselves. It must also be acknowledged in social and cultural spheres more encompassing than the self. We can glimpse the necessity for the public recognition and acceptance of a new body in the remarks of a professional woman describing how she explains MCS to others:

How I explain this illness to others depends first on how much time I have. If I only get a one-liner, I might actually say, inaccurately but usually effective, "Excuse me, but I'm allergic to your perfume or hair spray," for example. If there's a little more time, I'll say, "I have respiratory" (or "breathing") "problems which disallow any exposure to ambient chemicals.". . . If he or she inquires further, I explain, "I was poisoned by pesticides, asbestos, and other chemicals on several occasions. Having become chemically injured in this way renders me physically intolerant of chemical exposure." I might provide an example: "Right now your shaving cream and the moth balls in the closet sting me every time I inhale." The person will demonstrate a little shock, so I'll reassure him or her: "It's all right. Let's move over by the window. That will mitigate the effect." At this point, I may be asked to prove (though they'll never use the word) I was poisoned, or the nature of the injury. More frequently I am asked, "Well, what sorts of things bother you?" I reply that it is not a matter of anything "bothering" me, but rather, that various categories of chemicals cause me *pain*. Then I'll rattle off a list. I may also explain that I do not have to perceive any odor in order to be so affected, and will provide examples such as when, in a hospital just after a car accident, I was awakened from a double-dose morphine sleep by a spray of hair spray in the bed on the opposite side of a curtain in my room.

Sometimes people do want to understand better why those with MCS experience such pain and debilitation. With a highly educated person, I might present a combination of Bill Meggs's neurogenic inflammation" and Iris Bell's "limbic kindling" theories, leaning toward the former. Otherwise I might ask a person to imagine he or she had second-degree burns, internally, in the sinuses. "How might it feel," I ask, "if you were without functioning cilia—or any cilia at all, if your mucosa were dried and cracked, with several cell layers of damage, so that chemicals could easily eat into deep layers of sensitive tissue; and if someone then put a drop of iodine or chlorine or formaldehyde on that area? And what if this happened over and over, at every breath?"

If the inquirer can't understand intolerance of intermittent light, I explain that the electrical functioning of the brain depends on lipid-rich myelin sheaths surrounding nerves. Since there is an (autoimmune) antimyelin component to MCS, it could be that electrical impulses are more easily scattered. (This is upheld by gEEG studies.) Exposure to

EMR [electromagnetic radiation], including fields generated by fluorescent lights, could significantly affect brain electrical functioning where myelin is lacking. I present other reasons, too, with medical journal documentation, for why intermittent light may be deleterious.

Occasionally the listener needs to know prevalence, in which case I present the latest estimates that may be drawn from surveys by Bill Meggs, Iris Bell, and Claudia Miller. Usually these days, unlike at first, the listener will know someone who is chemically sensitive. "But he or she was also psychologically affected," I will often hear (which I take as a compliment). I then explain the difference between psychogenesis and the manifestation of psychological sequelae; and urge him or her to be careful not to be the judge. It is the case that people who have been told repeatedly by society that they are wrong, that they are mentally, not physically, ill, *will* begin to believe it—*and* to act that way. To presume mental illness of MCS sufferers in each case results in further physical injury (through lack of protection from chemicals), further disablement, and therefore further cost to society. It behooves society to presume physical illness just as in this democracy we are committed to presuming innocence, but with much higher stakes, in this case.

This thoughtful and detailed account hints at the importance of others to the ratification of a new body. In the following chapter we take up the issue of ratification, framing it as a problem of representation. If a new body is going to be more than a sociopsychological resource for the chemically reactive, it must be represented in reconfigured social relationships, new public and corporate policies, issues of litigation, and changes in the market, as well as, of course, sociological accounts such as this one. As we will see in the next two chapters, the environmentally ill body is carving out a quite visible, if still limited, presence in late modern society.

Part Three

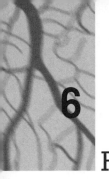

6

Representation and the Political Economy of a New Body

IMAGINE A SINGLE PERSON LIVING without the company of others who is free to exercise considerable control over his environments. Now suppose this person begins to experience frightening changes in his body as it touches or absorbs what were once thought to be safe places and things. A reasonable response to his dilemma would be a systematic inventory of his habitat to discover just what was making him sick. If in rearranging or changing his environments he also restored his health, this imaginary person could continue his life without devoting much additional attention to what originally troubled him.

Imagine this same person whose body is changing in relationship to local environments living in the company of others. He is married, has friends, works at a job, lives in a neighborhood, shops at local stores, and worships at a local church or synagogue. Now he must not only devise some scheme to control his symptoms; he must be prepared to explain his troubles to often skeptical others whose bodies routinely intersect local environments with no apparent injury or disability. He must acknowledge that what is an essential reality for him is likely to appear as sheer nonsense to many others, which is more than simply a communicative impasse because others must be willing to change to accommodate his troubled body.

In spite of the unusual nature of his somatic troubles, his rhetorical task would be considerably easier if he could invoke the authority of medicine to explain his body. Perhaps he is one of the lucky ones who encounters a sympathetic physician willing to believe the fantastic story he tells about his body. At least now he could ally himself with a professional, explaining his untoward symptoms in words beginning with "My doctor thinks I have . . ." The medical profession, however, is not likely to speak on his behalf. Typically, he must speak for himself, construct his own account of why he is sick, and convince others of its legitimacy.

If our account was limited to the first imaginary person, our story could have ended with chapter 5. It is, of course, this second—far from imaginary—person we must account for in this study. Success in convincing other people of the threat to health posed by mundane environments and ordinary consumer items is critical to the effective management of MCS. If a chemically reactive person is to live among others who are not multiply chemically sensitive, she must ask them to modify and change what have always seemed benign, if not aesthetic or pleasurable, behaviors; if they do not do so, they are implicated in the exacerbation of her illness. A spouse or lover, a friend, the checkout clerk at the grocery store, an office mate, a sociologist who requests an interview, and even a complete stranger become potential sources of acute, debilitating distress. The chemically reactive must approach each of these encounters armed with an explanation of their new bodies or must be prepared to retreat quickly to safer places. A bank teller remembers:

I knew I was going to have to tell my coworkers a convincing story the morning I wore a carbon-filtered face mask to work. My supervisor had agreed to let me wear it "on a trial basis," but she told me she would have to reassign me if it bothered the other employees. I practiced what I was going to say all the way to work.

In this short account, we see the need for the chemically reactive to negotiate new understandings and routines to survive in a chemically hostile world. Here the text of MCS becomes, in addition to a practical knowledge about the body, a type of "justificatory conversation" (Mills 1967), a rhetorical means to convince others to change or modify habits, routines, policies, and so on. To the degree people and policies change to accommodate the claims of MCS, a new body is being included, accepted, or, as Durkheim would say, represented in social and spatial configurations.

To narrate accounts of a new body is one thing; to get others to acknowledge such a body by changing personal habits, workplace policies, housing codes, manufacturing practices, and so on is quite another. But insofar as others do change in response to the needs of chemically reactive bodies, they are, whether intentionally or not, acting on behalf of a new somatic text. From changing something as personal as avoiding the use of a scented hair spray to rewriting a federal public housing code to accommodate the habitat needs of the environmentally ill, society is representing the existence of a new body. Insofar as these acts of representation become routine and expected, we can talk about the institutionalization of this body.

Chapters 3 through 5 have presented in detail the work of the chemically reactive to construct practical, useful accounts of the bizarre and frightening changes in their bodies. Working with the tools of rational inquiry and the symbols of biomedicine, they fashion interpretations of their immediate somatic and environmental experiences. In so doing, they are constructing a *model of* their misery (Geertz 1973, 93–94). A *model of* MCS permits them to grasp why and how the body is changing in relationship to environments. As a *model of,* MCS is a lay epistemology that works to render their misery comprehensible.

As a *model of,* a story about MCS told by a chemically reactive person corresponds closely to the classic idea of illness narratives, varying perhaps only in its unusual degree of medical elaboration. The word *illness* directs attention to the social and psychological experience of disease. Disease, falling squarely in the natural world, is the province of physicians. Physicians assign disease languages to bodies, and ordinary people experience their diseases as illnesses. At least that is how it is supposed to work. But the stories of the chemically reactive are more than illness narratives, more than subjective appraisals of discomfort, pain, and suffering; they are also explanations, answers to questions about bodies and environments.

They are not disease classifications either, at least in the conventional sense of originating from the medical profession. Environmental illness is not a *medical* disease, if the medical profession resists acknowledging it. Insofar as MCS is recognized by key social institutions, perhaps it is best thought of as a *sociological* disease. In other words, if key sectors of society respond to MCS as if it were a disease, it becomes, to paraphrase W. I. Thomas, a disease in its consequences. It becomes, in short, not only a *model of* a new body, but also a *model for* social change.

In this and the next chapter, we shift attention from MCS as a *model of* a new body to the more politically interesting question of MCS as a *model for* new social relationships, workplace regulations, public policy, and so on. Here EI becomes a disease theory wielded by nonphysicians that organizes social, political, and cultural spaces, fashioning them to represent a new body. Insofar as MCS becomes a *model for* new intimate relationships, friendship patterns, workstation norms, public health policies, litigation initiatives, federal housing codes, and so on, it becomes a political and economic reality in spite of its continual disavowal by the medical profession. If institutions routinely change in accordance with intelligence provided by legitimate arenas of technical expertise, in this case the amount of change occurring in response to an expertise wielded by nonexperts suggests a new type of institutional learning, one that acknowledges the political power of rational inquiry among laypersons.

In their work to make their bodies models for social order, the environmentally ill are engaging in what Giddens (1990) calls "life politics," or a "radical engagement" with others "to further the possibilities of a fulfilling and satisfying life for all" (156–57). After all, it would be difficult for the chemically reactive self (or any self, for that matter) to maintain indefinitely a nonrepresented or even an underrepresented body. For the environmentally ill body, symbolic and physical survival depends on the willingness and capacity of others to act as if MCS is a real medical disorder.

Writing as if he has the chemically reactive in mind, Giddens (1990) observes that to be political toward everyday life is to assume "an attitude of practical contestation towards perceived sources of danger" (137). To modify Giddens just slightly, it is the chemically reactive body that has an attitude, that contests through its somatic responses new, and previously unthought of, sources of danger. The self can be seen as speaking for this new "body with an attitude" using the sophisticated language of biomedicine.

The idea of the chemically reactive community engaged in life politics to secure social, cultural, and political recognition of the environmentally ill body is nicely illustrated in a document entitled the Declaration of Rights for Those with Environmental Illness. Embedding the life politics of MCS in the language of rights sounds a powerful and pervasive theme in American political philosophy. Recalling our discussion in chapter 5, the idea of rights is the centerpiece of the American justice system and a key to its expression of social consciousness.

Written by several prominent national advocates of the environmentally ill, including Earon Davis, Mary Lamielle, and Susan Molloy, the Declaration appeared in two nationally circulated newsletters in the late 1980s (*Delicate Balance*, March 1987; *The Reactor*, May–June 1987). Couched in the language of human rights to just and fair treatment, it demands the following:

- The right to competent medical practitioners with accessible facilities.
- The right to insurance reimbursement of expenses incurred in medical treatment and rehabilitation.
- The right to nondiscriminatory treatment in public and commercial buildings (including theaters, restaurants, stores, offices, recreation and spectator facilities) and public transportation through the removal of chemical and ventilation barriers to provide equal access and enjoyment.
- The right to nondiscriminatory treatment throughout the legal system, with the removal of chemical and ventilation barriers from courtrooms, hearing rooms, polling places, deposition locations, post offices, and other public places.
- The right to equal treatment from federal, state and local "entitlement" programs such as Social Security, Workers' Compensation, welfare, rehabilitation services, housing, etc.
- The right to reasonable accommodations in the workplace in order to reduce exposures for all of the public and to allow those who suffer from chemically/environmentally induced or exacerbated illnesses to remain employed. Such accommodations would include modifications to office environments through the removal or control of pollution sources and increased fresh air ventilation, changes in workstations, and work-at-home and/or part-time options.
- The right to protection from chemical exposures and the implementation of informational and protective systems throughout government and private industry to avert instances of "chemical trespass."

What is not said in this appeal to fair and just treatment is as important as what is said. By the time the Declaration was written, MCS was a fully developed lay epistemology. Susan Molloy, chemically reactive and one of the document's principal authors, is the editor of *The New Reactor* and organizer of the Environmental Health Network. She also earned a master's of public health degree at the

University of California, Berkeley, writing her thesis on MCS and access to public facilities (Molloy 1993). Earon Davis, an attorney and coauthor, works to get the language of MCS into the courts. He is the editor of the *Ecological Illness Law Report*. A third author, Mary Lamielle, has testified in federal congressional subcommittees on the environmental etiology of MCS. She was a principal witness in the hearing of the U.S. Senate Subcommittee on Indoor Air Quality Act in 1989, testifying to the etiology and identifying symptoms and consequences of MCS. Lamielle is the editor of the influential journal *Delicate Balance* and founder of the National Center for Environmental Health Strategies; she also is environmentally ill.

The language of rights to equal access, protection, respect, and entitlements, in other words, is based not simply on emotional appeals to justice but on the instrumental, rational knowledge of MCS as a legitimate medical disorder. In chapter 5 we argued that linking rights to instrumental rationality is an important modification in the struggle for social and cultural representation. Indeed, it is arguably a new expression of traditional political populism (see Couch and Kroll-Smith forthcoming).

In the next two chapters we use the ideas of MCS as both a *model for* a new body and a new life politics to examine the situated work of the environmentally ill to achieve a measure of cooperation from others. The idea of *others* can be placed in a rough order from immediate and intimate to secondary and abstract. Immediate others are those the chemically reactive know intimately: a spouse, a child, a friend. Such relationships are typically founded on emotive criteria and guided by a shared trust that each will treat the other with care and affection. At this elementary level, as we will see, it is more affective ties than lay epistemologies that shape the response of others to the chemically reactive.

At the next two levels, however, social recognition of MCS depends on the capacity of the chemically reactive to tell plausible, that is rational, stories about their bodies and environments. One level removed from the intimate is the world of secondary relationships negotiated between people and their employers, colleagues, fellow congregants, anonymous others, and so on. The environmentally ill encounter these more abstract others whenever they venture away from their families and friends. At its most abstract, the other is faceless, expressed in economic and cultural venues.

The importance of representation for a sociology of MCS cannot be underestimated. Representation, as Durkheim (1965, 462–96) was among the first to show, is a measure of how a society learns. At the abstract level of society, learning can be said to occur when collective practices and shared ideas change to accommodate claims made by interest or pressure groups seeking legitimation of their issues. Social change and institutional learning, in other words, are closely related.[1]

A notable achievement of modernity was to make scientific and communal ways of knowing incommensurable (Lyotard 1992; Touraine 1995). Thus modern societies typically learn in one of two fashions: from populist appeals to equality and justice, and from expert judgments about, among others, economic, legal, and medical orders of the world cast in languages of rational, instrumental knowledge. Contemporary societies, in short, are typically taught by two quite different mentors using two quite different didactic strategies: citizens, on the one hand, talking about their experiences and their rights, and experts, on the other, talking about experiments, statistical measures, and other indexes of instrumental rationality. And, not surprisingly, these two mentors often disagree with one another (Beck 1992; Touraine 1995).

The case of MCS, however, suggests a new pattern of institutional learning. Joining appeals to rights with claims to know something rational and thus real about bodies and nature, citizens are persuading institutions to change using two traditionally separate strategies. Ordinary people are using the complicated reasoning of medicine to argue for social and political recognition of a new relationship between bodies and environments. And they are arguing their case in opposition to many of the legitimate keepers of medical languages—physicians, medical researchers, and professional societies.

To the extent the practical epistemology of MCS finds representation among key social institutions, in spite of resistance among medical experts, it might be said we are witnessing a new form of social learning. Insofar as MCS becomes a model for secondary relationships, for public policies, for standing in courts of law, for commodity production, and for agreed-upon explanations of uncertain events, it can be said to be teaching society.

We start with a brief foray into the world of interpersonal relationships and close this chapter with an extended discussion of the relationships between ordinary people narrating complicated accounts of MCS and evidence of institutional change.

MCS and Primary Ties

The most immediate locale for the representation of the environmentally ill body is the intimate relationship or primary tie. Not surprisingly, stronger emotional attachments between people reduce the necessity to justify requests for change using complicated, technical narratives of somatic disorder. On the other hand, in the absence of strong primary ties, the use of biomedical narratives to justify change is not likely to prove effective. It is compassion, benevolence, and trust, not technical or rational knowledge, that are the keys to building and modifying intimate relationships. And of the three resources for building relationships, trust is arguably the most important in those cases where someone asks another to trust an account that cannot be easily verified. A dentist recalls his wife's response to his "long-winded account of the medical hocus-pocus of environmental illness. . . . 'I don't know anything about environmental sickness,' she said, 'but you look sick. What can I do?'"

Shared histories that create common ways of feeling and knowing make each participant a respected and trusted narrator in the "eyes of the other" (Giddens 1990). "Intimate others," as Giddens reminds us, are those "whose charity is forthcoming even in difficult times" (119). But, as we all know, this is an ideal, and rarely completely accurate, characterization of intimate relationships.

Evidence for change at this elemental level of social life is difficult to marshal into any kind of coherent story. Perhaps this is because the impetus or resistance to changing intimate relationships is based more on the pre-illness qualities of these relationships than on the problems of MCS itself. Unfortunately, we did not pursue this topic in our interviews with the chemically reactive. Nevertheless, we do have several accounts that illustrate the uneven and quite different outcomes that are likely to occur when a person asks an intimate other to accommodate a new and unusual body.[2]

For some people, their new bodies brought unexpected rewards in the form of stronger family ties. A professional woman who works as a manufacturer's representative writes: "My husband and I have actually become closer, more expressive, and more understanding of each other's needs. I have drawn closer to our daughters. They cared for me when I was at my worst."

A college professor and management consultant found her spouse distressed because of his limited ability to help: "My husband is as supportive as he can be—he is frustrated that he cannot help me. He does not want to think about moving to get away from the electric heat because gas is also not supposed to be good for MCS. It is very hard on him to see me in such pain and panic."

The concrete idea of representing the chemically reactive body at this intimate level of social life is nicely captured in the words of a chemical engineer: "My wife decided before I said anything about it to get rid of her perfumes, hair sprays, and so on. She told me, rather than me telling her, that they couldn't be good for me."

Family members who represent the environmentally ill body by making personal adjustments always do so at some cost to themselves. A producer and director writes:

> Andy has been extremely supportive. It was his urging and with his help that I got the disability pension. He follows my diet so we don't have to cook two meals. In some ways the MCS has brought us closer together, but in others it has created tension. Andy admits that he finds it frustrating not being able to make plans, as well as having to cancel

already made plans, depending on my condition. He also admits that it is difficult to live with someone who is chronically ill. He, too, is affected by the more isolated life we are now leading. . . .

Our daughter is very supportive. She seems to accept my illness, and indeed cannot remember a time when I was healthy. She shows only the occasional resentment of having more responsibilities around the house, and lives quite comfortably under all the strict rules about who and what can come into our home. Both she and Andy are very careful about not bringing anything in which might affect me and if they think that might be the case, they immediately change their clothes and have a bath.

In this passage we see how family members represent the body of the chemically reactive by changing their diets and social calendars, assuming additional domestic tasks, monitoring who comes into the house, and abiding by strict hygiene habits to prevent the outdoors from coming in. It is in these small but important ways that the environmentally ill body becomes a model for the family.

In addition to changing their personal habits and routines, some spouses and partners become social activists, representing the chemically reactive body to broader publics. A disability rights expert with MCS reports: "My boyfriend is usually very supportive. He tells his friends about my illness and my limitations. This is very helpful." A retired forestry executive writes about his wife: "Janice learned as much about MCS as I did and speaks to people about it. She gave a talk about chemicals and the body at our public library last month." Andy, the partner of the producer and director encountered above, "has always been a social and now environmental activist and often speaks out about MCS and its victims, especially in our present battle to keep chlorine out of our town's water system." An otherwise healthy person who identifies with MCS by advocating for its legitimacy as a real disease ensures the chemically reactive one more voice in their struggle for recognition.

Many of the environmentally ill, however, are not as lucky as these narrators. Indeed, the people who narrated their experiences to us report more failures than successes with representation at this basic level of human relationships. Trust is something like capital; it grows when wisely invested, and it can be lost if ill spent. But this analogy attributes too much agency to the self. In spite of someone's intention to build a relationship based on trust, trust requires the willing participation of the other. It is this immediate dependence on the other that makes it a form of social rather than economic capital. In the absence of trust, living with MCS is a difficult task indeed. A former professional musician who is now totally disabled writes:

> Neighbors and family were very critical; they were suspicious. They could see I was sick, but how could I react to something so severely, which didn't bother them at all? They thought it was all in my head. As a result, I lost contact with my entire family. My mother spread malicious rumors that it was psychiatric, and that ended my relationship with my sister, brother, aunt, uncle. I also could not very well show up and advocate for myself, since no one would cooperate with my needs.

The problem of trust, specifically a lack of it, is painfully evident in the remarks of a retired orchestra director:

> I was driven out of my family's home on account of chemical usage on December 31, 1984. My requests, then pleas, that they refrain from using fabric softener . . . perfume and hair spray and a kerosene heater went unheeded and eventually taunted. Friends didn't know what to make of me. They didn't "really" believe me.

Illustrating the idea of trust as a sum or quantity is a disabled teacher who can count on only her husband. She explains: "I have no relationships left except my husband. Never had any children. . . . The telephone is for emergencies, it never rings." A computer programmer writes, "My wife is my only friend. Even my kids have stopped coming around." A man who worked forty years with electrical cleaning solvents observes: "I can no longer work. My relationship with my wife seems much more strained. I used to belong to a veterans group—I was forced to quit due to the environment."

There are obviously significant variations in how family and friends respond to the need to accommodate the demands of a new and unusual body. Responses ranging from empathetic acceptance to cautious support to hostile rejection are based more on the relative presence or absence of trust than on the need to explain the chemically reactive body in rational, instrumental language. A general contractor with MCS recalls a conversation he had with his wife, who was suing for divorce after seven years of marriage: "I told her in detail about my illness and how it made me sick and all. She told me she understood all that, but had to leave anyway. I wasn't what she bargained for, I guess. . . . But you want to know something? I wasn't what I bargained for either." His wife claimed she understood his explanation of MCS, and the implication is that she accepted it. But she nevertheless walked out. At this level of human engagement, accepting the legitimacy of the MCS narrative is obviously not a condition for representing a new body. At the next, more abstract, level, however, to accept the authenticity of MCS is to be obligated to model public spaces, workplaces, churches, synagogues, and other built environments to reflect the special needs of this body. At this level it is not a question of liking or trusting as much as a question of agreeing that MCS is a legitimate physical disorder. Not surprisingly, it is in regard to secondary organizations and affiliations that a practical, rational, working knowledge of MCS must be persuasive.

Secondary Ties and Institutional Learning

The chemically reactive and their advocates are achieving some success in convincing their employers, city and county officials, and state and federal agencies to change or make policies that bear on the relationships of bodies to environments. The specific intersection between citizen accounts of biomedical changes in their bodies and institutional change is neatly expressed by Deloris, who finds her employer willing to accept her interpretation of the relationship of chemicals to the olfactory center of the brain: "I pointed to my nose and traced my finger from there to my brain and I explained that chemicals in my environment have damaged the sensory fibers in my cranial nerves." Apparently, her supervisor believed her account. Deloris is now permitted to wear a carbon-filtered mask at work when she detects untoward changes in her body.

Alan, a machine shop supervisor, tells his shop manager about chronic low-level exposures to PCBs and other chemicals found at the work site: "They are slowly but surely wearing down my immune system, reducing my ability to fight off colds, cuts, or scrapes and everything. I told him everything I was learning about MCS. He told me I sounded like 'a damn doctor.'" Alan's shop manager agreed to clean the work site ventilation system and maintain it according to standards set by the American Society of Heating, Refrigeration, and Air-conditioning Engineers.

While Deloris and Alan narrate accounts of specific changes in response to their lay epistemologies, illustrating the importance of ordinary persons wielding instrumental, rational accounts of bodies and environments, institutional change is also occurring in response to more concerted and collective efforts to educate the public. For example, the Labor Institute of New York, a labor advocacy group, published and distributed *Multiple Chemical Sensitivities at Work: A Training Workbook for Working People* (Pullman and Szymanski 1993). Its opening paragraph is revealing:

> Multiple Chemical Sensitivities (MCS)—a disorder caused by exposures to chemicals in the environment—has been acknowledged by very few in the medical profession. As a result, workers who are hyper-sensitive to chemicals in their workplaces are often viewed skeptically by their co-workers and ignored or harassed by their employers. (6)

The workbook is designed to help people with MCS narrate plausible and convincing accounts of their somatic reactions to workplace environments. Anticipating skeptical responses from employers and fellow employees regarding the reality of EI, it provides "factsheets" to challenge commonsense beliefs. For example, in response to the claim by a skeptical other that "chemicals . . . are adequately regulated by the government," the MCS advocate is directed to see factsheets titled, respectively, "The Health Effects of Chemicals Are Virtually Unknown" and "Protective Standards Not for MCS Sufferers."

"Activism 101: Ways to Educate Others about MCS" appeared in *Teach-In,* a journal published in Bellingham, Washington, and was adapted and reprinted in the July 1996 issue of *Toxic Times.* It addresses the importance of narration for the environmentally ill: "Each [MCS] sufferer can tell his or her story and make contacts. Individuals can write down their stories; they can assemble some current, significant information on MCS and turn it into an educational 'bridge-packet' for distribution to those who are ignorant about MCS" (8). The chemically reactive are advised, among other things, to

> share your personal story with anyone who is not familiar with MCS. . . . Write . . . your union and/or governmental agencies seeking their assistance in preventing further chemical injuries. Send them a "bridge-packet.". . . Volunteer to speak on radio talk shows, TV talk shows, or at educational meetings. . . . Become involved in legislative committee action. (8)

As if responding to the last recommendation, Lynn Lawson, who is chemically reactive and the editor of *CanaryNews Newsletter* of the Chicago-Area EI/MCS Support Group, reports testifying "at a local hearing of the National Institute for Occupational Safety and Health (NIOSH), one of three such meetings held across the country to obtain recommendations for that agency's research agenda for the next decade" (*CanaryNews* 1996, 2).

"EI activists" in New Mexico organized a

> fragrance-free Town Hall Meeting in Santa Fe to discuss the problems faced by chemically sensitive New Mexicans and to propose state level solutions. A panel of representatives from state agencies heard from EIers on the issues of housing, employment, health care. . . . The presentation opened the eyes of many state officials and furthered the process of securing recognition and accommodation in New Mexico. (*CanaryNews* 1996, 8)

Mary Lamielle, mentioned earlier in this chapter, regularly speaks for the environmentally ill body to authorities responsible for public health. Addressing a U.S. Senate Subcommittee on Superfund, Ocean, and Water Protection, she stated:

> People are becoming ill from the complex array of chemicals in building materials, furnishings, and consumer products. Some people with chemical sensitivity disorders become ill from a specific contaminant in the indoor environment. . . . many others have chronic exposures, a slow and subtle poisoning. . . . Symptoms from chemical sensitivity disorders include . . . fatigue, confusion, memory loss . . . seizures, and other neurological difficulties; respiratory involvement with bronchitis, asthma, and shortness of breath. . . . Many chemical victims must use activated charcoal filters or masks, respirators, or oxygen to minimize exposure. (U.S. Senate Subcommittee 1989)

Her testimony then segues into vignettes of people with MCS. For example: "A gentleman from Michigan developed multiple chemical sensitivities from exposure to vapors offgassing from a waterproofing compound applied to the basement wall." In 1989 several amendments proposed by Lamielle in this and other hearings were incorporated into Senate Bill 657, the Indoor Air Quality Act. A key amendment is her lay-expert definition of MCS: "The term 'multiple chemical sensitivities' describes an emerging syndrome characterized by a wide range of debilitating symptoms resulting from exposure to very low levels of several substances common to the typical indoor environment" (Amendments to "Indoor Air Quality Act of 1987," 1988/1989).

At a more local level, two MCS support groups, the Environmental Health Network and Health and Habit, persuaded officials in Marin County, California, to designate a small area in the courthouse off-limits to people wearing colognes, hair sprays, perfumes, and other scents offensive to the chemically reactive. While the success was a modest one (a row of folding chairs at the back of a public meeting room guarded by a sign designating it a fragrance free area), it is a good example of the redefinition of space to represent the chemically reactive body (*Delicate Balance*, spring/summer 1991, 14).

South of Marin County, the city council of Santa Cruz, California, passed a 1993 resolution entitled the Americans with Disabilities Act Self-Evaluation and Transition Plan. The plan was designed in part to protect the chemically reactive. Among its provisions are the following:

> a. remove chemical air "fresheners" from rest rooms and offices; b. switch to unscented soap in rest rooms; c. discourage the use of personal fragrances by City employees; d. no smoking in city vehicles, buildings, or the outdoor areas around building entrances or intakes; e. print on all City-sponsored event notices the following message: "Out of respect for those citizens with multiple chemical sensitivities, we ask that you attend the meeting fragrance and smoke free"; f. when possible use least-toxic products, maintain adequate ventilation when such products are used and signs of warning posted before, during and after such products are used. (*New Reactor*, 1994, 10)

Ecology House in San Rafael, California, is another example of representing the environmentally ill body at the community level. Its history is worth recounting. Before constructing an ecology house, the Public Research Institute at San Francisco State University needed baseline information on what constitutes a "safe house" for people with MCS. One hundred Bay Area residents who self-identified as multiply chemically sensitive were interviewed by telephone. They were asked to assess their tolerances to building materials, paints, carpets, furniture, and so on. Based on these data, a building profile was developed for construction of an eleven-unit, low-income apartment complex to accommodate individuals with EI and/or confined to wheelchairs. The "safe house," in other words, is a physical model of the environmentally ill body.[3]

A more momentous change is a law passed by the State of Washington on June 7, 1990. Pressed by several state organizations, including the Washington State Chemical Sensitivities Group, the legislature passed a bill requiring disabled parking privileges for those with "'an acute sensitivity to automobile emissions which limits or impairs their ability to walk'" (*Delicate Balance,* spring/summer 1990, 7). The law also mandates that people with MCS can drive up to the full-service pumps at gas stations and pay only self-service prices, thus protecting them from more immediate contact with gasoline fumes. This remarkable piece of legislation illustrates the capacity of the chemically reactive to successfully negotiate a medical determination of their problem in traditional political arenas, in spite of the medical profession's denial of the physiological basis of the disorder.

Representing the chemically reactive body in community initiatives and local and state ordinances is complemented by changes occurring in other organizational venues. A 1993 resolution by the National Association of Social Workers (NASW) delegate assembly, for example, recognized MCS as a disabling condition (Donnay 1996). Responding to the NASW's call to recognize the environmentally ill body, the University of Minnesota School of Social Work lobbied to create a "scent-free" safe zone for work and study to accommodate faculty, staff, or students who are chemically reactive.

The Methodist Federation for Social Action, a national group representing the United Methodist Church, adopted a resolution on indoor air pollution. The resolution urges local churches, church agencies, and institutions to

> invite those with special sensitivities to share the handicaps and suffering which they bear due to indoor air pollution, prohibit smoking in all indoor facilities, provide adequate fresh air ventilation, or high quality air cleaning equipment. If necessary, take an audit of sources of indoor air pollution and take remedial steps to correct the situation. (*Delicate Balance,* fall/winter 1989, 17)

The United Methodist Church's General Board of Global Ministries published an *Accessibility Audit for Churches,* which lists indoor conditions likely to make the environmentally ill body sick. It also offers suggestions on how to change the indoor environment to make it more safe for the chemically reactive (United Methodist Church, General Board of Global Ministries 1994).

The First Unitarian Society of Chicago organized an Environmental Task Force in 1995. Among the task force's objectives is to

> purchase, from now on, only those cleaners and other property maintenance products which are safe for people and the environment, in line with the [society's] Model Environmental Community Plan. . . . [This is done to recognize] the fact that our church has chemically sensitive individuals and should be open to others who are chemically sensitive. (Donnay 1996, 6)

Finally, the First Baptist Church of Houston, Texas, with a membership roll exceeding twenty thousand, established a "fragrance-free" Sunday school department and sets aside a "safe worship area" for the benefit of congregants with MCS (Donnay 1996).

Conclusion

Trust is a key to anticipating whether or not the chemically reactive body will be represented in primary, intimate ties; rational, instrumental knowledge, on the other hand, is a key to anticipating whether or not this body will find representation in more abstract secondary social and political ties. While we would not discount the importance of representing the environmentally ill body at the personal level of spouses, children, and friends, the problem of trust itself is linked to broader social and political patterns of rejection or accommodation.

A chemically reactive man is likely to find his family more accepting of his disability if his church or synagogue sets aside space for fragrance-free worship, if his employer cooperates in creating a safe space for him to work, and if an ordinance passed in his community recognizes the right of the chemically reactive to park in disabled parking places. Indeed, an argument could be made that with greater social and political representation of the chemically reactive body, a person will be less likely to have to rely on trust to secure understanding and assistance from family and friends. Trust will always be important in interpersonal relationships; it is simply made a good deal easier when what is at question is supported by broader, more inclusive social and political actions.

Changes in organizational behaviors, workplace policies, community ordinances, and so on, made to accommodate the chemically reactive body, suggest a practical observation: society does not always wait until the data document conclusively the presence or absence of a risk or hazard. Sometimes it acts with incomplete facts, uncertainties, and unknown consequences. In the case of MCS, society acts on the basis of an expert language wielded by nonexperts. Whatever changes an organization or community makes in the name of the environmentally ill body are made because this body is assumed to be physically real and not simply because employers, officials, and others are feeling kindly toward the chemically reactive. Instead, their practical theorizing about bodies and environments is influencing institutional others. A woman who identifies herself as chemically reactive writes, "I sound knowledgeable enough about the condition that most people take me seriously."

The next chapter continues our discussion of representation and social learning—first by linking MCS to several important pieces of federal legislation and to subsequent civil and tort litigation on behalf of the chemically reactive, and then by presenting evidence for the commodification of the chemically reactive body.

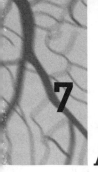

7

A New Body in the Courts, Federal Policies, the Market, and Beyond

If [a] plaintiff is successful in convincing a jury that the body's shield against the disease has been lowered, then only a handful of complaints over the plaintiff's lifetime may not be attributable to the chemical exposure. Therefore, the claim [of MCS] must be considered to be an extremely dangerous one in terms of the damage potential.

(Quoted in Bascom 1989, 35)

Legalizing the Multiply Chemically Sensitive Body

We can assume the term *damage potential* in the preceding is not referring to risk to human health and well-being but to the harm caused employers and manufacturers who must pay in the event they are found responsible for a plaintiff's physical disability. Recognizing the grave potential in legal recognition of MCS, the Chemical Manufacturers Association called for a coordinated effort between insurance companies, the medical community, and consumer product manufacturers to resist the definition of MCS as an environmentally induced disease (*Delicate Balance,* spring/summer 1990; spring/summer 1991). The concern is understandable.

Also understandable, though for quite different reasons, is the official recognition of MCS by the Association of Trial Lawyers of America (ATLA). In 1987 the Consumer and Victims Coalition Committee of the ATLA proposed a resolution acknowledging EI and supporting the rights of environmentally ill victims. The resolution was accepted by the general membership (*Delicate Balance*, March 1987). The ATLA reconfirmed its recognition of MCS as a litigative issue in its 1994 national meeting, referring to it as "an emerging and potentially major public health problem" (Donnay 1996, 10).

We need not question the motives of the ATLA in recognizing the environmentally ill body; the point is that it does. Moreover, plaintiffs' attorneys are assisted in their efforts to represent this body in the courts by two significant pieces of legislation: the Rehabilitation Act of 1973 and the Americans with Disabilities Act of 1990.

The Rehabilitation Act of 1973 prohibits discrimination against otherwise qualified persons with disabilities in any program or activity receiving federal funds, as well as in executive agencies and the Postal Service. The Americans with Disabilities Act (ADA) of 1990 states that reference to an individual disability means: "a. physical or mental impairment that substantially limits one or more of the major life activities of such individuals; b. a record of such an impairment; or c. being regarded as having such an impairment (42 USC, 12102, sec. 3).

Not surprisingly, the ADA is proving to be an effective resource for representing the chemically reactive body in courts. Its 1991 amendment, Regulation 1630, adds even more legal teeth to the ADA. Regulation 1630 requires employers to respond when employees report that one or more of their "major life activities," including walking, breathing, seeing, and hearing, are impaired by workplace conditions (*Americans with Disabilities Handbook*, 1991). This expanded definition of disabilities might seem to some people to have been written with the chemically reactive in mind. That is certainly the case with the New Jersey State Bar Foundation, which offers a toll-free phone number to order printed information about both the ADA and MCS.

Framing the chemically reactive body in the language of the ADA does more than expand a potential client pool, however; it shifts attention from the more limited medical model to the far more inclusive model of disability. Since disability is not limited to conditions of medical pathology, the chemically reactive are less dependent upon medical experts to confirm their practical ways of knowing the relationships between bodies and environments. They can move quickly from their often complicated lay epistemologies to the more obvious and easily documented problems of physical impairment in such critical life activities as breathing, walking, talking, thinking, and so on. Insofar as the issue of disabilities attends to function and not cause, representing the chemically reactive body is more a matter of documenting its impairments, a far simpler task than confirming a disease etiology or pathophysiology. Once disability is documented, the search for cause in the legal arena is far more flexible than a similar search in the medical arena, as the following two cases illustrate.

In *Kallas Enterprises v. Ohio Civil Rights Commission* (No. 14282, 1990 Ohio App. Lexis 1683 [Ohio Ct. App. May 2, 1990]), the Ohio Court of Appeals ruled the plaintiff was dismissed from the work setting illegally because of a disability. The appellate court upheld a lower court decision regarding "occupational asthma," finding that "hypersensitivity to [rustproofing] chemicals can be considered handicaps within the Ohio statutes for civil rights." The case begins with the civil issue of disability and ends with a legal recognition of handicap that includes hypersensitivity to rustproofing chemicals.

Similarly, in *Kouril v. Brown* (912 F. 2d. 971 [8th Cir. 1990]), the Eighth Circuit Court decided in favor of a woman who claimed to be disabled by MCS. Once her disabilities were documented, the court acknowledged their source: exposures to common chemicals such as ink, perfume, tobacco smoke, and odors emitted from photocopiers. In both of these cases we can see the courts applying a more flexible criteria of etiology than those typically employed by most physicians. Disability rights legislation is creating a back door, if you will, for legal—not medical—recognition of the lay epistemologies of the chemically reactive.

In addition to or in combination with the ADA, attorneys can also use workers' compensation laws to press for recognition of EI. Courts and workers' compensation boards in eight states have issued twelve separate rulings recognizing MCS as a physical disorder. In *Kehoe v. New Hampshire Department of Labor Compensation Appeals Board,* the New Hampshire Supreme Court found Denise Kehoe to be disabled by exposure to chemicals on her job site. Her symptoms include severe headaches, difficulty breathing, and allergies. The court decision includes the following legal endorsement for MCS: "[L]ittle doubt exists the multiple chemical sensitivity syndrome due to work place exposure to chemicals is an occupational disease compensable under our workers' compensation statute" (648 A. 2d 474 [N.H. 1994]).

In a second case a claimant is judged eligible to receive compensation benefits after it is determined that she is symptomatic only while at work. Chemicals offgassing from materials she works with, in combination with a warm temperature and poor ventilation, are determined to be the causes of her disability. According to the Oregon Court of Appeals, "she had shown by a preponderance of the evidence that the major contributing cause was her work environment . . . which exposed her to concentrations of chemicals much greater than she was ordinarily exposed to outside the course of employment" (*Robinson v. SAIF Corp.,* 717 P. 2d 1202–1206 [Or. Ct. App. 1986]).

A suit joining workers' compensation laws to negligence laws was brought against the Boeing Company. A unanimous decision by the Supreme Court of the State of Washington found in favor of the plaintiffs. The court found sufficient evidence that Boeing engaged in deliberate intent to do harm to seventeen of its employees, exposing them needlessly to dangerous chemical exposures. This ruling allowed the plaintiffs to sue for civil damages in addition to their workers' compensation benefits. The case was returned to a U.S. District Court and will be tried by jury (Supreme Court of the State of Washington, October 26, 1995, No. 62530-1).

More than a little irony is found in the negligence case of *Bahura v. S.E.W Investors* (1989). Several employees who worked on the third floor of the federal building housing the Environmental Protection

Agency claimed in a suit brought against the building contractors that formaldehyde offgassing from new carpet was the cause of mild to severe medical disabilities. The protectors of the environment themselves became victims of the spaces where work proceeds to protect the public. A jury found in favor of the plaintiffs.

If workers' compensation and negligence laws make it possible to represent multiply chemically sensitive bodies in workplaces, the Fair Housing Amendment Act makes it possible to represent them in domestic places. In fact, a right to adequate housing was originally a part of the first version of the Americans with Disabilities Act (West 1993). It was later deleted from the ADA, however, when legislators determined that persons with disabilities can appeal to the Fair Housing Amendment Act (FHA) of 1988. The FHA requires owners of public and private housing to provide adequate accommodations for people with physical disabilities (West 1993).

A letter from HUD'S assistant secretary written in 1990 makes it clear this federal agency recognizes the environmentally ill body as a "'disability entitling those with chemical sensitivities to reasonable accommodation under Section 504 of the Rehabilitation Act of 1973' as well as 'under Title VIII of the Fair Housing Amendment act of 1988'" (Donnay 1996, 6). This was followed in 1992 by a formal memorandum issued from the HUD deputy general counsel to all regional counsels stating that individuals disabled by MCS and EI can be handicapped within the meaning of the Act.

Attorneys writing for *Trial* magazine note:

> The conclusion that MCS can be a handicap under the FHA greatly helps people with MCS. The act provides them with a right not to be discriminated against because of their handicap when buying or renting housing. It also provides them with the right to an equal opportunity to use and enjoy their dwellings. (Lieberman, DiMuro, and Boyd 1995, 28)

Not only does the FHA work in the concrete manner just described to represent the environmentally ill body in domestic environments; it also affirms the existence of this new body, giving it a tangible legal identity. Joining the lay epistemologies of the chemically reactive to legislation and the courts bypasses the medical profession and expresses an alternative strategy for constructing a biomedical reality.

In *Lincoln Realty Management Co. v. Pennsylvania Human Relations Commission* (1991), Susan Atkinson filed a complaint against her landlord for failing to accommodate her physical disability. The commission summarizes her case:

> Lincoln ejected Atkinson from her apartment solely because of her physical disability, and rejected any reasonable accommodations she proposed in violation of the provisions of the Pennsylvania Human Relations Act. . . . Atkinson, who is extremely sensitive to a variety of chemicals and chemical products, entered into a one year lease beginning February 1986. By letter dated May 6, 1986, Lincoln informed Atkinson that her lease would not be renewed for the upcoming year as Lincoln was unable to provide her with the special treatment and precautions her condition demanded. Atkinson did not vacate . . . at the expiration of the lease term . . . and filed a complaint with the Commission. (598 A. 2d 594 [PA. Commw. 1991], 596)

The commission received her complaint and set a hearing date. At the hearing Atkinson testified she suffered from multiple chemical sensitivity.

> The hearing examiner found that Atkinson is handicapped within the meaning of the Act, that she established a prima facie case of discrimination, and that Lincoln did not make reasonable accommodations for her, and that Lincoln did not demonstrate that making reasonable accommodations imposed an unreasonable hardship. (598 A. 2d 594 [PA. Commw. 1991], 596)

The commission's judgment against Lincoln required the company to provide more effective ventilation of Atkinson's apartment (ceiling and exhaust fans); to use low-toxicity paints and pesticides; to provide two weeks' notice prior to painting, pesticide treatment, and lawn care; to use an organic lawn care program within a hundred-foot radius of her apartment; and to remove offensive floor covering and replace with it an acceptable material. The plaintiff is required by the commission to help pay for these changes.

In *Lebens v. Country Creek Association* (No. 94-940 A [E.D. Va. 1994]), Melinda Lebens filed a suit against her townhouse community association. She had asked the association on several occasions prior to the suit to implement an integrated pesticide management program in lieu of the usual blanket spraying. Rather than arguing its case in court, however, the association settled with Lebens, agreeing to pay a portion of her legal fees and to comply with the following changes: (1) eliminate blanket spraying programs for pests in the entire townhouse complex, including establishing a pesticide-free zone around her living unit; (2) identify and use chemicals that are low-level threats to Lebens along with mechanical and horticultural controls as alternatives to previous procedures; (3) provide seven days' notice prior to pesticide application and seek her counsel on which chemicals are the least dangerous to apply; (4) provide notice of planned new construction with potential chemical exposures and, again, seek her advice on how to minimize exposures; and (5) keep machinery away from her townhouse. In this example we see evidence of the chemically reactive body represented in corporate decisions about pest control and new building construction.

We do not know what proportion of legal cases involving MCS are decided in favor of the chemically reactive. Our intention is to provide sufficient evidence that the existence of a new body is recognized with some regularity in the deliberations and decisions of courts, commissions, and other legal venues. Joining the claims for a troubled body to disability, workers' compensation, and fair housing legislation in legal arenas would seem to suggest an alternative model for the public recognition of a disease, one that diminishes the role of medicine in the making of disease. It is as if the medical profession is on the sidelines watching a game between the chemically reactive and their attorney advocates on one side, and employers, landlords, and other responsible parties on the other side.

The marginal role of medicine in representing the environmentally ill body, while an important observation, is not a historical anomaly. Professional medicine has traditionally been reluctant to recognize diseases with environmental and occupational etiologies (Nelkin and Brown 1984; Freund and McGuire 1991). Coal miners and labor rights advocates, for example, knew well ahead of the medical community the devastating consequences of "black lung," or "miner's asthma" (Freund and McGuire 1991, 68). What makes MCS unique is the role of laypersons in fashioning rational, medical explanations for their subjective, somatic experiences. If a miner was likely to know a folk song about black lung, a person whose body changes uncontrollably in putatively benign environments is likely to construct an elaborate biomedical account of his misery. Perhaps this is because a lung disease caused by years of exposure to poorly ventilated, underground environments is an expected, if unwanted, occupational hazard, while a disease caused by routine exposures to culturally defined safe places requires thoughtful explanation.

Some occupational hazards, however, are not expected and are the source of considerable controversy. A legal contest involving the legitimacy of EI is currently being waged between the U.S. Veterans Administration and soldiers sent to Kuwait to fight the Iraqis. The action of the Gulf War was an intense, brief military and technological encounter that took place during the first two months of 1991. After limited occupation and little actual combat, U.S. troops returned home. Many men and women who had not come under enemy fire while in Kuwait and Iraq reported shortly upon returning home troublesome changes in their bodies, including aching joints, swelling of extremities, soreness, fatigue, memory loss, rashes, slurred speech, and loss of coordination (from President's Committee on Gulf War Syndrome 1995, cited in Parks 1996a).

A nationwide survey of 13,700 Gulf War vets conducted in 1993 by the Federal Department of Veterans' Affairs Persian Gulf Family Support Program found that 71 percent reported physical problems, including fatigue (25 percent), back, neck, and shoulder pain (25 percent), headaches (23 percent), skin rashes (18 percent), leg and arm problems (18 percent), stomach pain (14 percent), and breathing problems (14 percent) (Parks 1993b). Frank Bray, spokesperson for the regional office of Veterans Administration Affairs in Montgomery, Alabama, reports that claims by veterans for compensation almost doubled following the Gulf War, from 2,214 claims for the twelve-month period ending in February 1991 to 4,068 claims for the same twelve-month period in 1992–93 (Parks 1993a). In her oral testimony before the Committee on Veterans' Affairs, Subcommittee on Oversight and Investigations, on June 3, 1993, Dr. Claudia Miller of the University of Texas Health Science Center at San Antonio identified Gulf veterans as among the category of patients diagnosed as "chemically sensitive." Their bodies express typical MCS problems, including fatigue, numbness, dizziness, and headaches, associated with exposures to common, everyday chemical products and environments (U.S. House of Representatives Subcommittee on Oversight and Investigations 1993, 88). In the same hearing, Dr. Charles Henshaw, a physician with the American Academy of Environmental Medicine, concurred with Dr. Miller, noting, "The mysterious illness afflicting the Persian Gulf Veterans is multiple chemical sensitivity (91). To date more than twenty thousand Gulf War veterans have reported suffering from one or more of these symptoms (Parks 1996a).

In 1995 President Clinton appointed a citizen committee to review the circumstances and hear evidence regarding injuries caused by chemical exposures during the war. Recently a dozen ailing veterans from across the country represented their chemically damaged bodies to this committee. Nick Kresch, a thirty-year-old navy veteran, recalls his return from the Gulf War in 1991. At first he thought he had the flu, but the debilitating symptoms continued. His symptoms included weight loss (fifty pounds), bleeding from his gums and rectum, pain, and hair loss. "I got worse and worse," he explains, "and I worked less and less." After a series of downward events, he "hit bottom." He now receives full disability from the Veterans Administration and Social Security, but his symptoms persist (Parks 1996a).

Courts, congressional hearings, review boards, and other litigious settings will continue to be an important arena for dramatizing the problem of MCS. Defendants will continue to deny its legitimacy, while plaintiffs and their attorneys will work tenaciously to persuade judges and juries to recognize a new disease. At one, albeit abstract, level, social representation of the chemically reactive body does not depend on whether a particular case is won or lost. The fact that a case occurs at all means the question of MCS is a legitimate issue in civil, tort, or possibly criminal law. It is, perhaps, the nature of the legal profession to concern itself with a wider array of human troubles than the medical profession, which is limited to the problem of curing disease. For whatever reason, it appears the legalization of the chemically reactive body is occurring well ahead of its medicalization. Likewise, the environmentally ill body is being commodified faster than it is being medicalized.[1]

Commodifying the Environmentally Ill Body

Not surprisingly, the very market that produces consumer goods that allegedly cause or trigger MCS is also willing to produce goods targeted for the new needs of the environmentally ill body. Markets create consumers, openly and without apology. A television commercial that tells adults it is okay, if a bit naughty, to eat Kellogg's Frosted Flakes, is followed immediately by another commercial for Slimfast, a weight-loss product. And the irony is, few of us see the inconsistency of this juxtaposition of messages, encouraging high calorie consumption on the one hand and dieting on the other. We expect more honesty from ourselves and one another than we do from the market.

Ethical or not, however, markets in late capitalist societies are key resources for creating and representing cultural themes (Baudrillard 1975). To create a product is to also create a symbolic image of a consumer. A sixteen-bit True Value drill in a hard plastic case sitting on a hardware store shelf conjures up an image of a particular type of person, while excluding dozens of other types. When we see the drill, we are also likely to see this person, or could do so with little prompting.

The market, as we will see, is a key resource in both creating and representing the chemically reactive body. One carpet manufacturer participates in a program that seeks to "develop ways to reduce emissions by testing samples of carpet. With fresh air ventilation, most carpet emissions are substantially reduced within 72 hours after installation." In the same advertising statement the manufacturer also includes important health information, information for sensitive individuals, and carpet installation guidelines (*Delicate Balance*, fall/winter 1994).

One company, Pillows Futons Furnishings, offers a product list of items made with organic cotton. The advertisement, which appears in *Environ: A Magazine for Ecological Living and Health* (1994, 35), reads as follows:

- No pesticide, herbicide, or defoliant
- No flame retardant
- Fabric washed in filtered water
- All items made in a controlled air environment
- Packaged in cellophane

An ad in the same issue announces the Tenth Annual National Directory of Organic Wholesalers and Suppliers, noting that there are over eight hundred individually indexed commodities for the environmentally sensitive. In addition, a reader can purchase other indexes, which include "Buyers and Sellers of Every Kind of Organic Product, from across the US, Canada and Abroad." The directory cost $29.95 (33).

Specialty catalogues offer environmentally "safe" products. *Nontoxic Environments, Inc.* is an annual compendium of "building, household and personal products for the chemically sensitive and the earthwise." It is printed with soy-based ink on recycled paper. Among the items listed are safe home construction products: "Healthy Home Designs Portfolio: Environmental, Sustainable Architecture Designed for the Twenty-first Century"; "Eco Specs: A Guide to Planning,

Building, and Maintaining a Healthier Home"; Nilfisk GS Io commercial vacuum with felt microfilter and HEPA exhaust filter; Natural Linoleum; whole-house radiant ceramic heat; and portable, whole-house and auto air purification systems. Additional items include organic cotton pillows, Clearly Natural Soap, reusable menstrual pads, and a handmade face mask and filter in cotton or silk. The catalogue notes, "The products presented here are the safest alternatives we have found."

The Allergy Store in Sebastopol, California, offers a free sixty-four page catalogue of products proven effective for the sensitive person, which includes cosmetics, vitamins, air purifiers, household products, and much more.

The Living Source, a store in Waco, Texas, offers "products for the chemically sensitive and environmentally aware." Among the items on sale are ceramic, charcoal, and cotton masks; dental products for the chemically sensitive; deodorants for the chemically impaired; and "Denny Foil," a nontoxic substitute for tinfoil.

Cybertec, a cleaning franchise that specializes in services and solutions for sick building syndrome and indoor air pollution, advertises through the Internet. Another Internet entrepreneur advertises "new, affordable, disposable, activated carbon air filters—cure sick building syndrome by removing odors, molecular irritants and allergens, leaving indoor air truly clean and attractive."

If the courts are capturing MCS through what we might call the legalization of disease, the market is also claiming propriety over this nascent disorder. The chemically reactive body is quite obviously a market opportunity. Its peculiar needs are represented in product lines and services. Examine an activated carbon filter mask, a portable auto air purifying and circulation system, or a nontoxic substitute for tinfoil, and it is possible to discern the outlines of the chemically reactive body.

Commodifying the environmentally ill body is proceeding apace with legalizing it, while at the same time medicine continues to resist acknowledging it. This uneven institutional representation of this emergent body illustrates the idea that social learning is often fragmented, with one institution learning quicker than others and still others resisting, if not opposing, the lessons. The effects of this broken pattern of institutional learning on the self remain understudied, though we suppose they might create a more pronounced need for individual discretion than in situations where institutions agree.

Popular Culture and a New Body

A final, brief area worth considering is the representation of MCS in popular culture. Considered by some to be postmodern society's court of final appeal, popular culture is the most pervasive, some will say invasive, of our symbolic worlds. To be represented in popular culture is to exist, no matter how vacuous or empty the issue. The currently popular phrase "NO FEAR," for example, is found printed on clothing, stuck to cars, and tattooed on bodies, though its exact meaning, message, and origin are debated. As if conversing with or debating those who claim they are not afraid really mattered, the phrase "FEAR THIS" can also be seen on clothing, cars, and bodies. Indeed, T-shirts are available with one phrase on the front side and the other on the back. Insofar as popular culture enjoys the power to create and sustain essentially meaningless phrases, its authority over how we see and respond to our world should not be underestimated.

The popular television series *Northern Exposure* devoted several episodes to a young man who suffered from MCS. He lived in a bubble house, used a respirator when he ventured outside, and was an object of much scrutiny and conversation among his neighbors. Much to the chagrin of the chemically reactive community, however, he recovered from his disability when, of all things, he fell in love. Like the frog who is turned back into a handsome prince by the kiss of a princess, all you need is love to cure a debilitating environmental disease, or so the story goes. On the other hand, if the show's writers left the man disabled, they would also be required to write about the possibly toxic environments of a pristine Alaskan village, not a very upbeat theme for a feel-good series.

The chemically reactive body is also the subject of the recent movie

Safe. Set in Los Angeles, *Safe* is the story of a young, affluent house-wife who contracts MCS. It all starts when she and her husband buy a new house. Her body begins to respond to the paints, furniture, and new carpets in the house. She almost faints while driving behind a truck emitting carbon fumes from a faulty exhaust system. Her nose bleeds while she is visiting a beauty shop. Her symptoms persist, and her doctor recommends a psychiatric consult. The psychiatrist, a male, attributes her symptoms to stress caused by moving to a new neighborhood and house and counsels her to relax. She starts her own inquiry into her illness and attends a workshop on MCS.

Eventually, she separates from her family and moves into an alternative health community far removed from the city. The movie closes with her standing in the center of her one-room house, cot on the floor, a single lightbulb dangling from a cord attached to the ceiling providing the only light. She stares at an image of herself reflected in a small mirror hanging on the wall and whispers over and over again the New Age refrain, "I like you. I really like you."

Billed as a "dark comedy," *Safe* leaves the moviegoer wondering just what it was that made this woman so sick. Throughout the film she is depicted as unsure of herself, lacking a strong self-identity. The close of the film suggests she will recover from MCS when she begins to like herself. The source of MCS, in other words, is low self-esteem. On the other hand, the movie also makes it clear she is exposed to countless environmental insults. Perhaps the film is simply trying to be honest about this disease: there is a good deal we don't know about MCS.

Finally, a colleague who knew of our interest in MCS sent us the following poem by Alondra Orre, published in the February 1995 issue of *Blazing Tattles*, a monthly magazine with a focus on the political economy of environmental issues:[2]

Old MacDonald had a farm,
EI, EI, oh!
And on this farm was Pesticide,
EI, EI, oh!

With a spray, spray here, and a spray, spray there,
Here a spray, there a spray, everywhere a spray, spray
Old MacDonald had a farm,
EI, EI, oh!

The poem continues, replacing pesticide with fertilizer and antibiotics. It ends on the now familiar theme of lay inquiry.

Old MacDonald saw a doc,
EI, EI, oh!
The doc said, "It's all in your head,"
EI, EI, oh!
But he checked here, and he checked there,
Here he checked, there he checked, everywhere he checked, checked,
Till he found that he had got
EI, EI, oh!

To clarify for the reader, the publisher included the following postscript to the poem: "Publisher's note: 'EI' is an expression used to mean 'environmental illness' or 'multiple chemical sensitivity' (MCS)."

We do not have systematic data on how or how frequently popular culture represents the chemically reactive body, and anecdotes do not usually make a very convincing story. But we ask the reader to consider this brief foray into popular culture with the other evidence presented thus far to document the range of institutional settings that are recognizing a new body. And even without additional evidence of representation, we should not underestimate the role of popular culture in shaping attitudes, beliefs, and bodies in a culture oriented as much to symbols as to substance.

Conclusion

What changes when society recognizes MCS? Evidence presented in this and the previous chapter suggests the chemically reactive body is becoming a model for rethinking conventional boundaries between what is routinely considered safe and dangerous. If common understandings of safe and dangerous are important ways in which people acknowledge one another as members of the same society (Durkheim 1965; Douglas 1966), then each time the chemically reactive body is represented in some institutional context a new boundary between benign and perilous is drawn, however momentarily. People are invited to reconsider commonsense ideas about safe and dangerous. A portion of what everybody thought they knew with certainty is now a question.

AIDS, too, is a demand to revisit important life questions that appeared just a few years ago as manageable. Blood and sex—while always volatile cultural and biological issues—were thought to be under adequate control. Now, of course, we are not so sure. But whatever happens with AIDS, blood and sex will always be different from hair sprays and plastic wraps. We expect, or most of us do, that sustained attention is required to control the former, while the latter are, or were, until the emergence of MCS, thought to be comparatively safe. Environmental illness identifies nothing less than modern material culture as the source of debilitating disease. It is a way of explaining sick bodies that goes far beyond blood and sex, pointing its accusing finger away from the discrete person or couple to the world we have built for ourselves. "If a condom over my dick will protect me and my partner from AIDS," writes a young gay man with MCS, "then nothing less than a condom over all of my body will protect me from the environment."

The idea of representation invites consideration of how the lay theorizing of the chemically reactive is becoming a model for institutional practice. It allows us to complicate the orthodox perceptions of illness and disease by seeing how important institutional others respond to the definitional work of the chemically reactive not simply as a subjective experience of somatic distress but as a disease. Measures of this acceptance are found on a continuum from local, situated changes in workstation rules; to community and county ordinances; to federal legislation, the courts, and the markets; and to popular culture itself.

The case of MCS encourages us to be skeptical of the modern idea that physicians control the definition of disease while laypersons experience illness. The body of MCS, it appears, is protesting the conventional boundary between lay and expert medical knowledge.

~

The last five chapters have followed the narrative accounts of people who have constructed local, multidimensional classifications and conceptualizations of their bodies. Two assumptions guided our observations. First, we assumed that bodies exist before culture and in some fashion are always influencing human experiences. Second, we assumed that people are concept-creating and concept-bearing beings who will seek to comprehend and, if called upon, give an account of their bodies. In the case of MCS, we sought to show that knowing the body is necessary to both sociopsychological health and the well-being of the body.

From perceptions that something unusual is happening to their bodies to the development of rudimentary taxonomies of somatic signs and chemical agents, those with MCS are developing conceptual schemes for interpreting and coping with an array of unruly physical symptoms. They explain their rudimentary schemes to physicians, seeking confirmation and help. A few of the lucky ones are listened to by their doctors, and a kind of collaboration ensues between client and expert in a common cause to understand what is happening to the body. The majority of the chemically reactive, however, find their physicians unable, if not unwilling, to consider the validity of their emergent schemes associating physical symptoms with local environments and the chemical agents found in them.

Ignored or abandoned by their physicians, their symptoms persisting or growing worse, the chemically reactive construct their own biomedical accounts of what amounts to a new syndrome, if not a new disease. Separating the language of biomedicine from its institutional base, they transport it into their local worlds and fashion technical, some might say rational, accounts of their somatic troubles. Theorizing etiologies of disease that locate the source of affliction in subclinical exposures to putatively benign chemicals found in domestic, workplace, commercial, and other modern built environments, the nascent medical knowledge of the chemically reactive shifts attention from the body as a source of disease to the material world we all inhabit. Theorizing pathophysiologies of disease, the chemically reactive construct accounts, some quite elaborate, of the specific effects of chemical environments on a wide array of body systems, including respiratory, limbic, autoimmune, and nervous systems.

Borrowing from Geertz, we referred to these theories of MCS as lay epistemologies. In constructing biomedical accounts of their recalcitrant bodies, those with MCS are doing more than developing a practical approach to a practical problem; they are pointing to the possibility of a new way of knowing. Specifically, they are reclaiming the importance of subjective, human experience as a source of reliable, and rational, knowledge. Knowing, they contend, cannot be untangled from experience. Between the physical body and the environment is an active, conscious self ready to listen to the body as it encounters a world beset with peculiarly modern dangers. Joining the visceral knowledge of the body to the worlds of medical, toxicological, and ecological knowledge, the self fashions a reasonable account of physical distress and disability.

A rational knowledge that begins by paying attention to the language of the body and its relationship to environments might also assume that knowing is individual and local, indeed perhaps varying from body to body. An epistemology whose measure of reliability is biased toward the immediate, situated context challenges the classic assumption that reliable knowledge is universal, applicable to all people and all situations. The bodies of the chemically reactive can be likened to stations along the local train route. While the local stations are linked to one another by a common track, each one is individually named, acknowledging the particularity of place, and the conductor calls each station in turn. The MCS body is unique, separate from the other bodies, and requires explanation based on its particular, restricted relationships to immediate, tangible environments. On the other hand, it is linked to other bodies by a common thread of debilitating somatic responses to routinely benign places and commercial products.

Once biomedical language is used to explain the body and its strange relationship to environments, the validity of these explanations is more pragmatic and local than numerical and generalizable. A retired dentist who identifies himself as MCS put it this way:

> I know my explanation of MCS is correct because it works. It's as simple as that. I make better decisions with its help than I did without it. Maybe after all the research is in, if later someone locates my disease in my head and not my body and gives me a pill that cures me I'll believe his explanation. Until then I'm on my own.

Validity here is essentially a question of adaptation. Not "Is my explanation really true?" but "Is it practical and effective? Does my new knowledge of my body and environments help me adjust to, or survive, a world that is turned upside down, where safe has now become dangerous?"

We use the word *adapt* with caution. After all, if MCS is really a neurotic-somatizing disorder, lay theories of its environmental origin are themselves part of the problem. Perhaps the chemically reactive are constructing biomedical theories that are themselves nothing more than evidence of personality disorders. Luckily, we are not physical or biological scientists, and therefore can recuse ourselves from judging their accounts valid or invalid by the strict canons of science. We can offer a sensible observation on this question, however. If MCS is a neurotic-somatizing disorder, then we are witnessing the first recorded pandemic of people simultaneously expressing their neuroses through a critical assessment of somatic responses to local environments. From the village of Armidale, New South Wales, Australia, to Zurich, Switzerland, to the Black Hills of South Dakota in the United States, men and women, farmers, professionals, the young and the old are reporting their bodies changing in the presence of what are conventionally understood as safe places. And in the absence of a common organizational affiliation, they are constructing similar accounts of their troubles. It stretches common sense to write off this remarkable confluence of bodies, environments, and narratives as a psychiatric disorder prevalent throughout the world.

Another measure of the "truth" of MCS might be called sociological rather than clinical. Here and in chapter 7 we identified social, political, and cultural venues that are actively representing the chemically reactive body. If truth is a consequence of acting toward the world as if something exists, an increasing number of institutional others are making important adjustments to this new body and its theory of disease.

The final chapter expands our account of MCS to include another medical-environmental movement, popular epidemiology. It closes with several observations on environments, bodies, and rational knowledge.

Conclusion
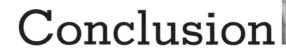

8

Bodies, Environments, and Interpretive Space

Proof is the bottom line for everyone.
(Paul Simon, "Proof")

IT IS A LATE SUMMER DAY in a southern university where a sociology professor is lecturing to a group of students. This class begins as others that preceded it during the semester, with nothing unusual happening. However, on this day, shortly after the lecture gets under way, two students in the back of the room begin coughing, making a dry, hacking sound. At first their coughing is barely discernible, but within a few seconds, several other students also start coughing. After a couple of more minutes, more students and then the professor are coughing. The classroom routine is disrupted. Something unusual is happening. The professor stops his lecture and asks the students what they think might be the source of their collective coughing. Several students said they detected a strong odor in the room, similar to the caustic smell of an institutional disinfectant. Within a few minutes the coughing subsides and class continues.

Did something in the air cause them to cough, or were they joined for a moment in a ritual of contagion, with one cough triggering another? The professor put this question to several students after class. For them, there was something in the air. He, too, admitted smelling something unusual in the classroom. They decided against the contagion theory and for an environmental explanation. Their collective decision to assume an environmental etiology, however, could be neither confirmed nor disconfirmed using standard biomedical models.

The amount of disinfectant in the room, assuming there was any, would in all probability fall well below the lowest-dose measure on any air monitor. And their unproductive coughs lasted only a few minutes, making them impossible to identify and track. A physician visiting the room within fifteen minutes of the incident might have heard a single cough throughout the rest of the hour—hardly reason to be concerned.

Incidents similar to the one described here appear to be occurring more frequently. While there are no reliable estimates of the number of such incidents, there is evidence that an increasing number of laypersons are assuming their bodies are somehow affected by ordinary, seemingly safe, environments. In his state of the world survey sponsored by the Gallup Institute, Riley Dunlap and his collaborators (Dunlap, Gallup, and Gallup 1992) found significant concern throughout the world, among poor and rich countries alike, for environmental degradation at local, national, and global levels.

He also found mounting concern for the deleterious effects of environmental problems on health. In 1982, for example, 27 percent of a random sample of British citizens believed their own health was affected a "great deal" or a "fair amount" by environmental stressors. By 1992, on the other hand, 53 percent of British citizens reported their health was adversely affected by environmental causes, an increase of almost 100 percent. Moreover, 79 percent of these same respondents believed environments would affect the health of their children over the next twenty-five years. The numbers in the United States also show a substantial increase in concern. Forty-five percent of a random sample of Americans reported the environment adversely affecting their health in 1982. By 1992 that number increased to 67 percent. Moreover, 83 percent of the U.S. sample believed the health of their children would suffer over the next twenty-five years because of environmental problems. Indeed, all of the twenty-two countries surveyed reported substantial increases from 1982 to 1992 in the number of people who believed their bodies were at risk of environmentally induced illnesses. Likewise, an average of 73 percent of respondents from all the countries surveyed believed environments would pose health risks for their children over the next twenty-five years (Dunlap, Gallup, and Gallup, 1992). Most people, it appears, believe that as environments become increasingly disorganized, so do bodies.

As publics become more concerned with health and environmental pollution, however, biomedicine is having an increasingly difficult time explaining bodies and the despoiling of nature. It is almost as if conventional biomedical theory and practice are marching off in one direction while bodies are marching off in the opposite direction. The growing space left between bodies and biomedicine is creating room for—more appropriately, the necessity for—lay interpretations. The problems of environments and bodies are opening up interpretive spaces for popular or lay expertise in what are otherwise closed worlds of professional judgments. Consider the role of interpretation in the professions.

Interpretive Space

The modern means of social control, Foucault (1977) argued, is not physical force but the application of cognitive rationality to physical, psychological, and social problems. It is the authority of rational knowledge exercised through the professions, not the threat of violence, that organizes, classifies, and explains bodies, selves, deviance, environments, and so on.[1] Social order is achieved through the careful management and application of specialized, technical knowledge.

But social and political power does not accrue to just any type of rationality (Turner 1995). A systematized and routinized knowledge, while not without its own capacity to control (a point made time and again by Weber) is less powerful than an expert knowledge based on a degree of indeterminacy. The one requires simple application, while the other requires considered distinctions among conceptual possibilities (133). It is not the routine application of technical knowledge that creates authority but the subjective expertise of the professional elucidating and explaining the relationship between abstract principles and concrete, empirical problems. The prestige of medicine as a profession is based in part on the generous space allowed physicians for the art of interpretation. The space between medical knowledge and somatic troubles cannot always be filled by the application of routinized knowledge. Sometimes this space calls for discerning, conceptualizing, and theorizing possibilities. A rough correlation exists between the need for interpretation and the amount of authority exercised by a profession.[2]

We agree with Turner and others on the importance of interpretive versus routinized knowledge to the exercise of professional power, though we argue by way of conclusion that expert interpretations themselves are rarely serendipitous but follow well-worn paths carved out by the paradigms of the professions. If expert interpretations are going to succeed as sources of social control, however, they must at some level satisfy the rational, emotional, and somatic criteria of the individuals and groups to whom they are applied. Otherwise they must be enforced through means other than their own internal claims to know. Consider, for example, citizens who do not accept the results of a government study that finds land adjacent to their community an "environmentally safe" location for storing low-level radioactive waste. Popular rejection of government and corporate science might force authorities to switch from control through the velvet glove of social and environmental impact studies to the stick of imminent domain law to secure the site.

Ironically, while biomedicine is considered one, if not the, most powerful profession, it is arguably most susceptible to popular resistance. Ultimately, biomedicine must make sense of the body—if not to heal it, at the very least to explain it to the layperson in some reasonable fashion. While the self might be a purely social construct, the body will always be, in part, natural and organic, outside the reach of social fabrication. Bodies, in short, can and do resist professional interpretations. They may respond in ways that elude cures, as in the case of AIDS or drug-resistant tuberculosis, or they may signal the need for altogether new ways of thinking about bodies, as in the case of MCS.

Modern bodies and their problems with environments are disorganizing the conventional relationships between laypersons and experts and are revealing a growing conflict between professional knowledge and the knowledge of ordinary people. Professional medical knowledge increasingly imposes dense, incoherent interpretations of bodies troubled by their immediate physical environments. When somatic states resist the domain assumptions of biomedicine, an interpretive space is created for the self who must continue to live with a body whether or not physicians, epidemiologists, risk assessors, and others can explain it.

Complicating and extending this idea, we suggest that it is not only the singular environmentally ill body that is challenging the hegemony of expert systems; it is also the more abstract populations of bodies represented in controversies over citizens and epidemiologists, toxicologists, and other experts. At issue in these conflicts are reliable and valid criteria for determining disease clusters and exposure rates in communities allegedly affected by toxins. In both individual and community cases, the subjective experiences of somatic conditions and environments can be neither confirmed nor explained using professional biomedical models.

Popular Epidemiology and the "Bio-politics of the Population"

Foucault (1979) examined in some detail how the modern state defined and controlled both individual bodies and populations of bodies, referring to the former as the "anatomo-politics of the human body" and the latter as the "bio-politics of the population." If the singular bodies of the MCS are important evidence for a growing disjunction between biomedical models and somatic misery, their problems are complemented by more abstract communities of bodies who are also increasingly forced to recognize the limits of state-sponsored medicine. Consider the following two cases, beginning with the well-known drama at the Love Canal.

Love Canal

The New York Department of Health (DOH) believed the chemicals buried under a middle-class housing tract in Niagara Falls were spreading uniformly throughout the neighborhoods. Working from this assumption, the DOH conducted a health effects study based on concentric rings radiating from the buried chemicals. Working from a different assumption, homemaker and emerging grassroots activist Lois Gibbs worked with a couple of her neighbors to survey residents in the subdivision. She found clusters among families whose houses sat atop dry underground streambeds, or swales.

> I knew of one swale, an old stream bed that went behind my house. I drew that swale on the map. Later, I drew a swale that Art Tracey, Mary Richwalter, and some of the other old-time residents had told me about. Actually, my neighbors drew the line for the swales. I was surprised: the illness clustered along the swales. (Gibbs 1982, 66–67)

Taking her observations to public officials, she was ridiculed and her results dubbed "silly housewife data."

Convinced she was on to something, however, Gibbs approached biologist Beverly Paigen with her numbers; together they developed the "swale hypothesis," which predicted that contamination was carried by water through these swales and therefore posed more danger to people living along the swales than to people who lived closer to the dump (Levine 1982, 87–94). This hypothesis was later confirmed by the Environmental Protection Agency.

Herbicide 2,4,5-T

In 1980, Britain's National Union of Agricultural and Allied Workers (NUAAW) was disputing a government regulatory decision to allow the use of the herbicide 2,4,5-T (Irwin 1995). The defoliant's potential hazards included spontaneous abortion, chloracne, and birth defects. Britain's Advisory Committee on Pesticides (ACP) argued that the defoliant "'offers no hazard' to users or the general environment 'provided that the product is used as directed'" (Irwin 1995, 19). To counter the ACP's conclusion, the NUAAW conducted its own studies. A survey of members registered the many difficult conditions a person was likely to operate in while preparing and using an herbicide. It asked people to assess the quality of safety and use information accompanying the chemical compound. Finally, it asked respondents to identify physical signs and symptoms they had experienced while using the herbicide. Surveys of similar medical problems in other countries were included. In addition to the survey, twelve illness histories were compiled of people who became sick while using the compound.

With its own database in hand, the NUAAW asked the ACP to consider an alternative strategy for assessing the risks of 2,4,5-T. Specifically, it argued for the need to use a "balance of probabilities" logic in judging the risks involved in using 2,4,5-T. The NUAAW's experiences of the compound, systematically compiled and reported, linked to data on application in other countries, and illustrated by a dozen concrete case studies, were, it argued, sufficient evidence to doubt the safety of the product (Irwin 1995, 114).

~

These two examples illustrate another movement wherein ordinary people are appropriating techniques and concepts from an expert system, joining them to their personal experiences, and petitioning in a language of instrumental rationality for institutional recognition of their troubles. In both the Love Canal and the 2,4,5-T controversies, health assessments conducted by laypersons were joined with their direct experiences of the hazards to contradict officially sponsored studies or force recalcitrant agencies to respond to locally perceived health problems.

Sociologist Phil Brown calls this specific movement "popular epidemiology." This variant of the medical science concept of epidemiology provides both a critique and a reorientation of the term. According to a standard medical textbook, "Epidemiology studies the distribution of a disease . . . and the factors that influence this distribution. These data are used to explain [disease] etiology [and recommend] preventive . . . practices" (Lilienfeld and Lilienfeld 1980, 4). Lay involvement in epidemiological research is discouraged for fear of biasing procedures (Freund and McGuire 1991).

In contrast to the traditional definition of epidemiology, Brown (1992) defines popular epidemiology as

> the process by which laypersons gather scientific data . . . and marshal the knowledge and resources of experts in order to understand the epidemiology of disease. . . . it emphasizes social structural factors as part of the causal disease chain . . . and challenges basic assumptions of traditional epidemiology, risk assessment, and public regulation. (269)

Captured in Brown's provocative definition is the idea that methods and concepts of traditional epidemiology are borrowed from the expert system and transferred to lay or nonexpert systems, thus shifting the social location of theorizing the origin and distribution of morbidity and mortality. With popular epidemiology the locus of knowledge shifts decidedly away from the expert system of medicine toward the grassroots and begins with situated experiences.

Importantly, following her experiences at Love Canal, Lois Gibbs did not return to her homemaker role. She moved to Washington and started the Citizens' Clearinghouse for Hazardous Waste (CCHW). Since its founding in 1982, the CCHW has helped over seven thousand grassroots groups cope with the problems of contamination, political organizing, and health. The organization has produced over sixty manuals and handbooks (Everybody's Backyard 1996, 3). Included among the titles are "Medical Waste" and "Common Questions about Health Effects." There is a manual, complete with questionnaires, on how a community group can do its own health survey. There are also "fact packs" of news articles on epidemiological subjects, including "Cancer Clusters," "Dioxin Toxicity," and "Lead Toxicity."

Often aided by social movement organizations and their allies, communities are encouraged to collect and analyze their own health data. The Environmental Health Network, a national grassroots organization, is currently conducting popular epidemiology studies in more than a dozen communities affected by hazardous waste problems throughout the United States (EHN *Newsletter* 1992). Another organization, Citizens Urge Rescue of the Environment (CURE), seeks to join the experiences and ideas of communities concerned with the distribution of disease and pollution with the more abstract knowledge of academics. It seeks to build locally based understandings of health problems and industry and to educate others. Its mission statement captures the organization's intentions clearly: "Our goal is to bring about awareness of the dangers of chemicals that produce various cancers . . . and remove them from use. . . . Since 1983 C.U.R.E. has carried this grassroots message to universities, governments, [and] grade schools as requested."

The change in social location represented by popular epidemiology is not always a complete rejection of experts. Indeed, it is a good example of how experts themselves can be appropriated by nonexperts. Some licensed experts become attached to environmental movements and community groups, lending technical knowledge and legitimacy to the popular epidemiological perspective. What is important from our vantage point, however, is that in those instances where experts align themselves with citizens, the citizens acquire both the knowledge and its embodiment, the expert, thus appropriating and controlling two important rational knowledge resources. Brown (1992), for example, notes the cooperation between a citizens' group (whose independent neighborhood health surveys suggested a link between water contamination and leukemia) and scientists at the Harvard School of Public Health: the citizens "no longer had to seek scientific expertise from outside; now they were largely in control of scientific inquiry" (271).

Citizens in control of epidemiological studies are likely to expand the circle of culpability to include purportedly safe environments typically ignored in government-sponsored research. Popular epidemiology ascribes to a view of evidence that expands the idea of dangerous or risky environments. It is considerably more flexible than traditional epidemiology in setting standards for proof that call for remedial actions (Recall the NUAAW's "balance of probabilities" argument). According to Brown (1992), traditional epidemiologists "prefer false negatives to false positives—i.e., they would prefer to claim falsely that an association between variables does not exist when it does than to claim an association when there is none" (274). In contrast, Linda King, the director of the Environmental Health Network, argues that epidemiology, like clinical medicine, should be committed to "false positives, that jargon that means the environment is considered dangerous until it is proven that it's not" (EHN *Newsletter* 1992).

Proponents of popular epidemiology argue that even without statistically significant data one can find satisfactory association between contamination and health problems across persons, places, circumstances, time, and so on (Brown 1992; Irwin 1995). Other proponents argue that circumstantial evidence should be considered valid: "Not every person who gets sick near a hazardous waste site gets sick *because of* the waste in the site. Yet very often there is strong circumstantial evidence to corroborate residents' beliefs that illnesses derive from toxic exposures" (Lewis, Keating, and Russell 1992, 4).

Finally, the toxicological question—What level of exposure is toxic?—is answered in a seemingly reasonable, if unconventional, manner in a paper prepared by the CCHW:

> One part per million means that there is one milligram of that substance for every kilogram of body weight. For . . . an adult weighing 59 kilograms (130 pounds), a dose of 1 ppm equals 59 milligrams. The average aspirin contains 325 milligrams of active ingredient, so that two tablets would be approximately the equivalent of 11 ppm in a 130 pound adult. This dosage can stop pain and reduce fever. [Thus] 11 ppm could mean a lot to the human body. (Lester and Gibbs 1988, 15)

Defining proof in the logics of false-positives, satisfactory associations, and circumstantial evidence, while linking toxicity levels to comparisons between toxins and aspirin, is likely to implicate a much broader number of environments and environmental agents in accounting for disease origins. Similar to the knowledge claims of the chemically reactive, popular epidemiology medicalizes the modern biosphere, expanding the number of local environments that are considered toxic and the source of disease.

Shifting the social location of epidemiology from professional to lay communities and expanding the possibilities for identifying correlations between environments and disease is creating a struggle over who will control the privilege to officially define the boundaries between safe and dangerous environments. Among the more prominent salvos in this skirmish is a report issued by the Environmental Health Network and the National Toxics Campaign that uses the principles of popular epidemiology to critique the traditional epidemiology of the federal Agency for Toxic Substances and Disease Registry (ATSDR) and the Centers for Disease Control (CDC).

The report refers to government-sponsored health studies as "inconclusive by design" (Lewis, Keating, and Russell 1992) and quotes researcher-activist Beverly Paigen, who claims that the ATSDR and the CDC "feel as if public hysteria is the most feared thing, rather than actual serious health effects. So they are always minimizing the effects" (12). In response to this report and the media attention it received, the CDC and the Environmental Protection Agency conducted a workshop in the summer of 1994 in Annapolis, Maryland, to determine more effective ways to include communities in environmental medicine research.

Evidence for the recognition of the persuasive use of epidemiology by the nonexpert community is also found in technical agency acknowledgment of the "health assessment review process." Organized by the Environmental Health Network, this process subjects agency health studies to critical review based on the principles of popular epidemiology. A personal letter to the director of the Michigan Department of Public Health from the Families for Environmental Health Awareness (a regional popular epidemiology group) notes that "health studies issued from your agency will be carefully reviewed by our health assessment staff. This strategy was used in Louisiana and in every instance where communities followed-up with public health officials [*sic*] data their demands were met."

The evidence for the social representation of popular epidemiology in public policies, agency-sponsored research protocols, and so on is not yet well developed. However, these examples point to its influence in suggesting new standards for proof and holding technical agencies accountable to rational accounts of bodies and environments put forth by nonexperts.

~

Thus, it is not just the singular bodies of the MCS that are falling outside the halo of biomedical explanation; whole populations of bodies reporting symptoms in relationship to environments remain unaccounted for using standard biomedical models. Popular epidemiology is a contemporary medical movement that seeks to expand the amount of interpretive space people in neighborhoods and communities can exercise in determining the relationships between patterns of morbidity and environments.

Environmental illness and popular epidemiology invite us to examine the boundaries between bodies and environments as sites of considerable controversy and equivocation. Modern bodies, it appears, are telling us that many contemporary illnesses are as much ecological as medical. But MCS and popular epidemiology are not simply citizen replications of bioscience models; rather, they represent alternative forms of rational knowledge constructed by people whose bodies no longer conform to the underlying assumptions of orthodox medicine. Ordinary people are fashioning a new form of rationality to account for changes in their bodies, blurring the boundaries between layperson and expert.

The Fall of Dualisms

A principal axiom of modernity was the separation of lay and expert knowledge. Lay knowledge was to be narrative in character (Lyotard 1992). It would concern itself with practical and emotional stories about how to organize one's life, how to fall in love, how to mourn, how to be a parent, and so on. Against this customary knowledge, however, would be the abstract knowledge of experts. Expert knowledge would be scientific, with its claim to truth resting exclusively on tangible and measurable proof. It would name things in the universe and show empirically how they are related. (Recall our account of the father and his newborn in chapter 2.)

If narrative knowledge creates and sustains community, scientific knowledge can be said to discover the patterns and laws of nature. The two ways of knowing could not be farther apart. Narrative knowledge begins with human experiences, while scientific knowledge begins with experiments. Narrative knowledge is eclectic, drawing from biographical experiences, the experiences of others, imagined experiences, and so on. Scientific knowledge, on the other hand, is anything but eclectic, requiring meticulously followed research designs that routinely include a rigorous defense against the intrusion of narrative knowledge.

Like similar dualisms that served to organize modern life—mascu-

line-feminine, subjective-objective, universal-particular, and so on—
narrative and scientific knowledge were to be conceptually and
socially distinct (Lyotard 1992). The history of modernity might be
read as a moment in time when bipolar, complementary ways of being
and knowing structured human life. Contemporary history, however,
invites a different reading; it appears to be a time when dualisms are
collapsing.

The boundaries between masculine and feminine are breaking
down as "transgendered" people claim a political space of their own
between men and women (Goldberg 1996). Thomas Kuhn (1970), a
physicist, admitted the importance of subjectivity in the allegedly
objective vacuum of science. The feminist movement forced us to
acknowledge that the "personal is political," joining the particular to
the universal. In each of these changes in interpretation, what were
once distinctly separate strategies for organizing society are now, if
not indistinct from one another, sufficiently blurred to suggest a new
history.

Multiple chemical sensitivity and popular epidemiology are ways
of knowing bodies and environments that join narrative knowledge to
biomedical knowledge, confounding yet another important dualism in
modern life, creating what we might call a popular or civic rationality.
A popular rationality begins with local experiences that require
understanding. Its form of reasoning recognizes that "consciousness
will never be sovereign over experience" (Frank 1995, 143) but that
reasonable, purposive action might follow from acknowledging their
importance to one another. Its problems are experiential, and its
responses are argued to be in accord with reason.

Puzzles, Mysteries, and Popular Rationality: Revolution or Reform?

Popular rationality has always been with us, of course. It is a
historically important mode of human adaptation, preceding institutional science and its handmaiden, technology. Before the grand nar-

ratives of science, practical problems were often successfully addressed through a combination of folklore or local knowledge, sensible planning, and most probably a fair measure of good fortune. Knowledge was contextual and local, resting on the simple assumption that knowing something important about nature could not be sequestered from mundane experiences. Knowing, in other words, could not be "disembedded from 'living'" (Irwin 1995, 122). But that, we are told, was long ago.

Modern societies reject both the importance of situated experiences and the people who have them in favor of a professional science that is at once self-generating, self-controlled, and self-regulating. In this society, personal experiences will always be secondary to the pronouncements of state-sponsored sciences. This is not to say, however, that all that is said in the name of science or enlightenment is necessarily believed. Recall Bolingbroke's observation on Descartes's hypotheses about animals: "The plain man would persist in thinking that there was a difference between the town bull and the parish clock" (quoted in Thomas 1983, 35). But while "plain men" could choose to believe their eyes despite what a scientist "knows," their sensate knowledge and experiences must be kept strictly separated from the laboratory or experiment. As any undergraduate methods book will advise, subjectivity must be rigorously precluded from entering scientific discourse lest it "contaminate" the conversation.

The benefits of a society administered by experts and expert knowledge rather than physical violence should be self-evident. Rather than threatening or hurting people to get them to cooperate, modern society could demand respect on the less painless claim to know far more than the average person about the order of society, the natural world, bodies, and so on. It was rational, scientific knowledge, not violence, that secured common purpose and encouraged a view of modernity as more civilized than "less modern" times and places.

But like all forms of authority, "rule by reason" must enjoy sufficient legitimation to sustain its privileged place. The authority of modernity depended in part on its capacity to transform mysteries into puzzles (Frank 1995, 80–81). Its calculus for accomplishing these transformations was, of course, the administration of expert knowledge organized to discover generalizable laws about the universe. Mystery is anathema to science because it admits of no solution; puzzles, on the other hand, invite them.

It was Kuhn (1970) who alerted us to the sleight-of-hand technique regularly used by science to ensure that the problems it examined were of a kind to admit of puzzles rather than mysteries—to wit, its reliance on paradigms or models that are both ways of seeing problems and ways of not seeing them. Kuhn writes, "One of the things a scientific community acquires with a paradigm is a criterion for choosing problems that . . . can be assumed to have solutions" (35). It is true, of course, that in the world of the laboratory or clinic, as Kuhn made clear, the paradigms of biology, physics, chemistry, and biomedicine regularly find relationships that, according to their logics of explanation, should not exist. These surprises, aptly called "discoveries," prompt a rethinking of an existing paradigm or a shift to a new paradigm altogether. The point for us is that these machinations are typically accomplished behind closed doors, out of sight of the public. Even the adoption of a new paradigm, what Kuhn calls a "scientific revolution," is a quiet rebellion fought in the civil confines of professional meetings and on the pages of arcane scientific publications. In Kuhn's work we can find the seeds for a critique of how real problems can remain nonissues. Its reliance on paradigms "insulates the [scientific] community from . . . socially important problems that are not reducible to the puzzle form because they cannot be stated in terms of the conceptual and instrumental tools the paradigm supplies" (1970, 37).

If the scientific community does not in general concern itself with social problems, it eagerly pursues solutions to production problems. The paradigms of science are routinely created and deployed to further the ends of capital production and are likely to systematically ignore its environmental, medical, and social consequences. Production is a scientific puzzle, while most of the effects of production remain mysteries.

Powerful interests in modern society want to know more about how to produce than about the "external" costs of production (Schnaiberg 1980, 277). Funding production science has always been a higher priority than funding impact science. Thus it should come as no surprise to learn that paradigms of production far exceed paradigms of impact in both number and sophistication (Schnaiberg 1980; Beck 1992). Sociology itself can be understood as contributing to the theme of production science. Parsons's seminal work (1951) on the sick role is a construction of the interaction between patient, family, and physician designed to return the sick person to work as soon as possible.

An increasing number of contemporary bodies, however, are protesting capital production, allegedly made sick from working in offices, factories, and schools, or simply living in putatively safe neighborhoods and communities. But not only is producing a capital goods society a source of disease; consuming the goods produced is also putting bodies at risk. The problems of MCS and popular epidemiology express the idea that the production of both bodies and environments is in conflict with the modern production of capital. Marx was perhaps the first to recognize this conflict. He theorized, some would say idealized, the rise of a rebellious working class that would claim its right to collectively own the means of capital production. But Marx wrote about a different time. To his credit, however, there is a rebellion of sorts. It is not a violent protest, as Marx predicted, but a cognitive one.

But it is not the cognitive conflict Kuhn describes. It is, rather, a third type of conflict. It begins with a narrative knowledge of bodies and environments—akin to Marx's emphasis on material conditions—and joins this knowledge to borrowed languages of expertise to construct new paradigms of knowing not envisioned by Kuhn or Marx.

Marx and Kuhn, of course, wrote about revolutions, albeit in quite different contexts. Environmental illness and popular epidemiology are not revolutionary, although they do call for significant social changes. The two movements are more reformist in orientation. They are best viewed as collective bargaining tools for individuals and groups who seek public recognition of their miseries. Their successes are good examples of how liberal democracies are amended and reformed, securing change while simultaneously affirming the authority of what Douglas and Wildavsky (1982) call "the center" of society, a hierarchical arrangement that seeks to perpetuate itself by "avoiding turbulent social processes" (92–93). Although social and political recognition of citizen expertise might be a cause of grave concern to some experts, their concern is based not on a popular cry to dismantle the system but on a request to more fully participate in it. It is the status of an expert or two that may be at risk, not the significance of expertise to social order.

In a society organized around reformist, progressive traditions, achieving meaningful social change is more likely to occur through successfully manipulating the languages of "the center." Popular rationality is a grassroots claim to understand important things about the world based on an interaction between narrative and scientific ways of knowing that is at once sensible, reasonable, and just. It is an important contemporary ingredient of the American reformist tradition and is likely to become more important to a society increasingly organized around the identification and management of environmental risks. Indeed, the incapacity of normal science to reach consensus on the scope and severity of complex, uncertain biospheric dangers is becoming apparent to an increasing number of people (Beck 1992). The cacophonous voices of experts, combined with the high medical and social stakes in identifying and managing these new dangers, are forcing an increasing number of ordinary citizens to theorize their bodies and environments for the practical purpose of securing a modicum of safety and well-being.

Environmental illness and popular epidemiology are not modern incidents of hysterical contagion or "cancer-phobia," as many have claimed, though evidence of social suggestion and fear can be found in each movement. They are evidence of an important untapped resource in contemporary society: the body and the reasonable, knowledgeable self inhabiting it.

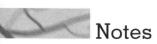 Notes

Notes to the Introduction

1. A point nicely made by Arthur Frank in his valuable book *The Wounded Storyteller* (Chicago: University of Chicago Press, 1995).

Notes to Chapter 1

1. It is worth noting, however, that if EI is an anomaly for biomedicine, it is a tangible expression of the truth claims of a marginal and disputed body of medical knowledge commonly called *clinical ecology* or *environmental medicine*. Clinical ecology is not recognized by the American Medical Association, in part because it assumes people can be made sick by ordinary environments, particularly petrochemical exposures. It is our impression, however, that comparatively few people who self-identify as environmentally ill have ever heard about clinical ecology, though they may learn something about it as they read, conduct research, and conceptualize their somatic troubles. (On the comparative insignificance of clinical ecology for EI, see Kroll-Smith and Ladd 1993.)

2. Illustrations like Ann's appear throughout this discussion. They are taken from newsletter accounts and interviews. Our research methods are explained at the end of this chapter.

3. To facilitate discussion, we will not always refer to both environments and products as sources of distress. When we use the word *environment,* we are implying both setting and products.

4. It is obvious to us, and we hope to the reader, that the demographic mix and areal distribution of people who claim to be environmentally ill suggest an organizational form considerably more complicated than a cult.

5. While no one disputes its commitment to rationality, it is doubtful the modern period will be remembered as a historical epoch guided by sensibility and wisdom.

6. To anticipate some semantic confusion over the words *epistemology* and *theory,* we are using the term *epistemology* to mean the nature of knowl-

edge. Environmental illness is a way of knowing that combines abstract biomedical concepts with concrete, local, somatic experiences. The term *theory,*
on the other hand, refers to the specific accounts of the environmentally ill
who use biomedical knowledge to explain their somatic distress. Taken
together, the theories of the environmentally ill constitute a practical epistemology, a way of knowing their bodies and environments based on biomedical nomenclature. If epistemology means *how* one knows, theory means
what one knows.

Notes to Chapter 2

1. The keystone assuring the hegemony of medicine was set in place at
the turn of the twentieth century, when the power of the medical institute was
firmly locked into the process of social control. It was in the "promise" of certainty offered by the medical community to render understanding of human
suffering and an offer to employ medical expertise in the resolution of this
suffering that a deal was made. Under the leadership of the American Medical
Association, the medical community offered its expertise to the state in
exchange for power and control (Starr 1982).

2. This is one dimension of Parsons's "sick role" (1951, 428–47). Not
surprisingly, the environmentally ill want very much to be recognized as sick,
but on terms considerably different than Parsons envisaged. For the chemically reactive the issue is not simply a temporary exemption from normal role
requirements but also a need to reconsider the requirements themselves. If
working with fax and copying machines is making an employee sick, then
modifying work routines might be necessary to accommodate him.

Notes to Chapter 3

1. Our thanks to Susan Kroll-Smith, who suggested a comparison
between Kafka's *Metamorphosis* and the problems of being environmentally
ill.

Notes to Chapter 4

1. Note, we are not saying that the chemically reactive believe their bodies exist independently of their emotions, or, for that matter, their brains. But
they would argue vehemently against the idea that their thought processes
could create their illnesses.

2. Remember, however, our sample is not random. Perhaps people who
self-selected to participate in our interviews did so in part to express anger at
the medical profession.

3. It is true, of course, that physicians are aware that cigarette smoke, perfume, and strong soaps, for example, may increase the discomfort of asthma patients. But "few physicians . . . would view these irritants as a primary cause of their patients' asthma" (Ashford and Miller 1991, 9). Biomedicine is also quite able to account for acute exposure to toxins. At issue here are nonacute, chronic, low-level exposures.

4. Our source for the following discussion of bodies and germs is Emily Martin's remarkable book *Flexible Bodies* (1994). See in particular part 2, "Historical Overview." See also Martin 1990.

Notes to Chapter 5

1. Those with MCS are not without their allies in the academy. A small group of philosophers, anthropologists, and others also grant the body a voice in the determination of social and political relationships (Sheets-Johnstone 1992; Locke 1993; Martin 1990; Frank 1991).

2. Kirmayer suggests that "aching bodies remind us there are at least two orders of experience: the order of the body and the order of the text" (quoted in Lock 1993, 142).

Notes to Chapter 6

1. Irwin (1995) argues expansively for this position in his book *Citizen Science:* "The concept of 'social learning' implies that this level of institutional change may be one of the most valuable of science-citizen encounters" (140).

2. And, we would add, this is a topic that deserves considerable attention as chronic, unexplained illnesses increase in number.

3. Representing the chemically reactive body in houses is recognized as a market opportunity by specialty builders like Darlene Cornelius Lowell, who is identified in *Our Toxic Times* as being "interested in building housing for MCS sufferers." Relationships between MCS and the market are discussed in the following chapter.

Notes to Chapter 7

1. The concept of medicalization is, in our opinion, more politically interesting when it is separated from its origins in labeling theory and considered both as a rhetorical resource for nonphysicians and as a process of institutionalization that competes with other corporate interests to capture a problem.

2. We thank Professor Craig Harris, Department of Sociology, Michigan State University, for sending us this poem.

Notes to Chapter 8

1. Readers can test themselves to see if they have internalized the authority of the medical profession by recalling occasions when they felt they *should* see a doctor or advised others to do so. And for those readers who have ever felt a bit guilty because they avoided a visit to the doctor, the proof of this profession's authority is in the feeling.

2. For a good discussion of the identity problems of pharmacists, who are increasingly defined as pill dispensers and businesspeople and less as professionals responsible for esoteric knowledge, see Turner 1995, 139.

Bibliography

Ad Hoc Committee on Environmental Hypersensitivity Disorders. 1985. "A Report to the Minister of Health." Toronto: Office of the Minister of Health.

American Academy of Allergy and Immunology, Executive Committee. 1989. "Clinical Ecology." *Journal of Allergy and Clinical Immunology* 78:269–71.

American College of Occupational Medicine. 1990. "ACOM Adopts ACP's Position on Clinical Ecology." *ACOM Report,* September, 1.

American College of Physicians. 1989. "Clinical Ecology." *Internal Medicine* 3:168–78.

Americans with Disabilities Act of 1990. PL 101-336. Title 42, USC 12102 et seq: *U.S. Statutes at Large* 104:327–78.

Americans with Disabilities Act Self-Evaluation and Transition Plan. 1993. NS21, 285. Santa Cruz, CA: City council.

Americans with Disabilities Handbook. 1991. Published by the Equal Employment Opportunity Commission and the U.S. Department of Justice. Washington, DC: U.S. Government Printing Office.

Ashford, Nicholas, and Claudia S. Miller. 1991. *Chemical Exposures.* New York: Van Nostrand Reinhold.

Atkinson, Paul. 1995. *Medical Talk and Medical Work.* London: Sage.

Bammer, Gabriele, and Brian Martin. 1992. "Repetition Strain Injury in Australia: Medical Knowledge, Social Movement, and De Facto Partisanship." *Social Problems* 39:219–37.

Bascom, Rebecca. 1989. *Chemical Hypersensitivity Syndrome Study.* Baltimore: Maryland Department of the Environment.

Baudrillard, Jean. 1975. *The Mirror of Production.* St. Louis: Telos Press.

Bauman, Zygmunt. 1993. *Postmodern Ethics.* Oxford: Blackwell.

Beck, Ulrich. 1992. *Risk Society.* London: Sage.

———. 1995. *Ecological Enlightenment.* Atlantic Highland, NJ: Humanities Press.

Berger, Peter, and Thomas Luckmann. 1966. *Social Construction of Reality: A Treatise on the Sociology of Knowledge.* New York: Anchor.

Bickerton, Derek. 1990. *Language and Species.* Chicago: University of Chicago Press.

Black, Donald W., Ann Rathe, and Rise B. Goldstein. 1990. "Environmental Illness: A Controlled Study of 26 Subjects with '20th Century Disease.'" *Journal of the American Medical Association* 264:3166–70.

Bond, J., and S. Bond. 1986. *Sociology and Health Care.* Edinburgh: Churchill Livingstone.

Brodsky, Carroll. 1984. "Allergic to Everything: A Medical Subculture." *Psychosomatics* 24:731–42.

———. 1987. "Multiple Chemical Sensitivities and Other 'Environmental Illnesses': A Psychiatrist's View." *Occupational Medicine: State of the Art Reviews* 2:695–704.

Brown, Phil. 1992. "Toxic Waste Contamination and Popular Epidemiology: Lay and Professional Ways of Knowing." *Journal of Health and Social Behavior* 33:267–81.

———. Forthcoming. "Popular Epidemiology Revisited." In special issue of *Current Sociology: Toxic Contamination and Community Transformation,* edited by Stephen R. Couch and Steve Kroll-Smith.

Brown, Richard, and Paul R. Lees-Haley. 1992. "Fear of Future Illness, Chemical AIDS, and Cancerphobia: A Review." *Psychological Reports* 71:187–207.

Bullard, Robert D. 1990. *Dumping in Dixie.* Boulder: Westview.

Burke, Kenneth. 1973. *The Philosophy of Literary Form: Studies in Symbolic Action.* Berkeley: University of California Press.

———. 1989. *On Symbols and Society,* edited by Joseph Gusfield. Chicago: University of Chicago Press.

Calhoun, Craig. 1995. *Critical Social Theory.* Oxford: Blackwell.

California Medical Association. 1986. "Clinical Ecology: A Critical Appraisal." *Western Journal of Medicine* 144:239–45.

Carson, Rachael. 1962. *Silent Spring.* Boston: Houghton Mifflin.

Chemical and Engineering News. 1994. "Facts for the Chemical Industry." June, 25–30.

Chemical Manufacturers Association. 1994. Trade advertisement.

Commission for Racial Justice, United Church of Christ. 1987. *Toxic Wastes and Race in the U.S.: A National Report on the Racial and Socio-Economic Characteristics of Communities with Hazardous Waste Sites.* Cleveland: United Church of Christ.

Conrad, Peter, and Joseph W. Schneider. 1990. *Deviance and Medicalization: From Badness to Sickness.* St. Louis: C. V. Mosby.

Couch, Stephen R., and Steve Kroll-Smith. 1994. "Environmental Controversies, Interactional Resources, and Rural Communities: Siting versus Exposure Disputes." *Rural Sociology* 59:25–44.

———. Forthcoming. "Environmental Movements and Expert Knowledge: Evidence for a New Populism." *International Journal of Contemporary Sociology.*

Crumpler, Diana. 1990. *Chemical Crisis: One Woman's Story.* Sydney, Australia: Scribe.

Cullen, Mark. 1987. "The Worker with Multiple Chemical Sensitivities: An Overview." *Occupational Medicine: State of the Art Reviews* 2:655–61.

Davidoff, Linda. 1991. "Multiple Chemical Sensitivity: Research on Psychiatric/Psychosocial Issues." Paper presented at Symposium on Multiple Chemical Sensitivity, American Public Health Association, Atlanta, Georgia.

———. 1992. "Models of Multiple Chemical Sensitivities (MCS) Syndrome." *Toxicology and Industrial Health* 8:229–47.

Davis, Earon S. 1986. "Ecological Illness." *Trial,* October, 33–34.

"Declaration of Rights for the Multiple Chemically Sensitive." 1981. *Delicate Balance,* March.

DeHart, Roy L. 1995. "Multiple Chemical Sensitivity: What Is It?" In *Multiple Chemical Sensitivity: A Scientific Overview,* edited by Frank L. Mitchell, 35–39. Washington, DC: U.S. Department of Health and Human Services and ATSDR.

Denzin, Norman. 1993. *Symbolic Interactionism and Cultural Studies.* Oxford: Blackwell.

DiGiacomo, Susan. 1992. "Metaphor as Illness: Post-modern Dilemmas in the Representation of Body, Mind and Disorder." *Medical Anthropology* 14:109–37.

Donnay, Albert. 1996. *Recognition of Multiple Chemical Sensitivity.* Baltimore: MCS Referral and Resources.

Dossey, Larry. 1984. *Beyond Illness.* Boulder: New Science Library.

Douglas, Mary. 1966. *Purity and Danger.* London: Routledge and Kegan Paul.

———. 1973. *Natural Symbols.* New York: Vintage Books.

Douglas, Mary, and Aaron Wildavsky. 1982. *Risk and Culture.* Berkeley: University of California Press.

Dubos, René. 1959. *The Mirage of Health.* Garden City, NY: Doubleday.

Duehring, Cindy, and Cynthia Wilson. 1994. *The Human Consequences of the Chemical Problem.* White Sulphur Springs, MT: Chemical Injury Information Network.

Dumont, Louis. 1986. *Essays on Individualism: Modern Theory in Anthropological Perspective.* Chicago: University of Chicago Press.

Dunlap, Riley E., George H. Gallup Jr., and Alec M. Gallup. 1992. *The Health of the Planet Survey.* Princeton, NJ: George H. Gallup International Institute.

Durkheim, Émile. 1965. *The Elementary Forms of Religious Life.* New York: Free Press.

Engle, George L. 1977. "The Need for a New Medical Model: A Challenge for Biomedicine." *Science* 196:4286.

Environ: A Magazine for Ecological Living and Health. 1994. No. 14.

Environmental Health Network. 1992. *Newsletter.* Great Bridge Station: Chesapeake, VA.

"'Environmental Illness' Briefing Paper." 1990. Washington, DC: Chemical Manufacturers Association.

Epstein, Steven. 1991. "Democratic Science." *Socialist Review* 21:35–63.

———. 1995. "The Construction of Lay Expertise: AIDS Activism and the Forging of Credibility in the Reform of Clinical Trials." *Science, Technology, and Human Values* 20:408–37.

Figlio, Karl. 1978. "Chlorosis and Chronic Disease in 19th-Century Britain: The Social Constitution of Somatic Illness in a Capitalist Society." *International Journal of Health Services* 8:589–617.

Foucault, Michel. 1973. *Birth of the Clinic.* London: Tavistock.

———. 1977. *Discipline and Punish.* London: Tavistock.

———. 1979. *The History of Sexuality, Vol. 1.* London: Allen/Lane, Penguin Books.

Frank, Arthur. 1991. "For a Sociology of the Body: An Analytic Review." In *The Body: Social Process and Cultural Theory,* edited by Mike Featherstone, Mike Hepworth, and Bryan S. Turner, 37–102. London: Sage Publishers.

———. 1995. *The Wounded Storyteller.* Chicago: University of Chicago Press.

Freund, Peter E. S., and Meredith B. McGuire. 1991. *Health, Illness and the Social Body.* Englewood Cliffs, NJ: Prentice-Hall.

Geertz, Clifford. 1973. *The Interpretation of Cultures.* New York: Basic Books.

———. 1983. *Local Knowledge: Further Essays in Interpretive Anthropology.* New York: Basic Books.

Gibbs, Lois Marie. 1982. *Love Canal: My Story.* Albany: State University of New York Press.

Giddens, Anthony. 1990. *The Consequences of Modernity.* Stanford, CA: Stanford University Press.

———. 1991. *Modernity and Self-Identity.* Stanford, CA: Stanford University Press.

Goldberg, Carey. 1996. "'He' 'She' They fight for Respect." *New York Times,* September 30.

Gordon, Deborah R. 1988. "Tenacious Assumptions in Western Medicine." In *Biomedicine Examined,* edited by M. Lock and D. R. Gordon, 19–53. Boston: Kluwer Academic Publishers.

Gusfield, Joseph. 1963. *Symbolic Crusade.* Urbana: University of Illinois Press.

Habermas, Jurgen. 1968. *Toward a Rational Society.* Boston: Beacon Press.

Harvey, David. 1989. *The Condition of Postmodernity: An Enquiry into the Origins of Social Change.* Oxford: Blackwell.

Hileman, Betty. 1991. "Chemical Sensitivity: Experts Agree on Research Protocol." *Chemical and Engineering News,* April 1. Washington, DC: American Chemical Society.

Indoor Air Quality Act of 1989. U.S. Senate Sub-Committee Hearings on Environmental and Public Works (S. Hrg. 101–2). Washington, DC: U.S. Government Printing Office.

Irwin, Alan. 1995. *Citizen Science.* London: Routledge.

Jewett, Don L. 1992. "Research Strategies for Investigating MCS." *Toxicology and Industrial Health* 8:175–79.

Jewett, Don L., George Fein, and Martin H. Greenberg. 1990. "A Double-Blind Study of Symptom Provocation to Determine Food Sensitivity." *New England Journal of Medicine* 323:429–33.

Johnstone, Albert A. 1992. "The Bodily Nature of the Self or What Descartes Should Have Conceded Princess Elizabeth of Bohemia." In *Giving the Body Its Due,* edited by Maxine Sheets-Johnstone, 16–47. Albany: State University of New York Press.

Kafka, Franz. 1972. *Metamorphosis.* New York: Bantam Books.

Kahn, Ephraim, and Gideon Letz. 1989. "Clinical Ecology: Environmental Medicine or Unsubstantiated Theory." *Annals of Internal Medicine* 111:104–6.

Kozak, David. 1994. "Reifying the Body through the Medicalization of Violent Death." *Human Organization* 53:48–54.

Kroll-Smith, Steve. 1995. "Toxic Contamination and the Loss of Civility." *Sociological Spectrum* 15:377–96.

Kroll-Smith, Steve, and Anthony Ladd. 1993. "Environmental Illness and Biomedicine: Anomalies, Exemplars, and the Politics of the Body." *Sociological Spectrum* 13:7–33.

Kuhn, Thomas. 1970. *The Structure of Scientific Revolution.* Chicago: University of Chicago Press.

Lawson, Lynn. 1993. *Staying Well in a Toxic World.* Chicago: Noble Press.

Lester, Steve, and Lois Gibbs. 1988. *A Citizen's Guide to Risk Studies.* Arlington, VA: Citizens' Clearinghouse for Hazardous Waste.

Levine, Adeline G. 1982. *Love Canal: Science, Politics, and People.* Lexington, MA: Lexington.

Lewis, Sanford, Brian Keating, and Dick Russell. 1992. *Inconclusive by Design.* Harvey, LA: Environmental Health Network.

Liberman, Michael S., Bernard J. DiMuro, and John B. Boyd. 1995. "Multiple Chemical Sensitivity: An Emerging Area of Law." *Trial*, July, 22–33.

Lilienfeld, Abraham, and David Lilienfeld. 1980. *Foundations of Epidemiology.* New York: Oxford University Press.

Lock, Margaret. 1993. "Cultivating the Body: Anthropology and Epistemology of Bodily Practice and Knowledge." *Annual Review of Anthropology* 22:133–55.

Lyotard, Jean-François. 1992. *The Postmodern Explained.* Minneapolis: University of Minnesota Press.

Martin, Emily. 1987. *The Woman in the Body.* Boston: Beacon Press.

———. 1990. "The End of the Body." *American Ethnologist* 19:121–40.

———. 1994. *Flexible Bodies.* Boston: Beacon Press.

Mastermind, Margaret. 1970. "The Nature of a Paradigm." In *Criticism and the Growth of Knowledge,* edited by I. Lakatos and A. Musgrave, 59–89. Cambridge: Cambridge University Press.

Mead, George H. 1967. *Mind, Self and Society.* Chicago: University of Chicago Press.

Mills, C. Wright. 1967. "Situated Actions and Vocabularies." In *Symbolic Interaction: A Reader,* edited by Jerome G. Manis and Bernard N. Meltzer, 335–68. Boston: Allyn and Bacon.

Minor, Mary. 1994. "*Comments on Public Health Assessment, Keystone Sanitation Landfill, Hanover, Adams County, Pennsylvania,*" CERCLIS NO. PADO54IRS781, November 10.

Mitchell, Frank L., ed. 1995. *Multiple Chemical Sensitivity: A Scientific Overview.* Washington, DC: U.S. Department of Health and Human Services and ATSDR.

Molloy, Susan. 1993. "Measures Which Will Result in Greater Access for People with Environmental Illness/Multiple Chemical Sensitivity to California's Public-Funded Facilities: Steps toward Regulatory Remedies." Master's thesis, University of California, Berkeley.

Nash, Roderick. 1989. *Rights of Nature.* Madison: University of Wisconsin Press.

National Academy of Sciences. 1987. *Workshop on Health Risks from Exposure to Common Indoor Household Products in Allergic or Chemically Diseased Persons.* Washington, DC: National Academy Press.

National Research Council. 1991. *Environmental Epidemiology: Public Health and Hazardous Wastes.* Washington, DC: National Academy Press.

National Research Council's Board on Environmental Studies and Toxicology. 1992. *Report.* Washington, DC: National Academy Press.

National Research Council's Board on Environmental Studies and Toxicology, Committee on Neurotoxicology. 1994. *Models for Assessing Risk, Environmental Neurotoxicity.* Washington, DC: National Academy Press.

Needleman, Herbert L. 1991. "Multiple Chemical Sensitivity." *Chemical and Engineering News,* June 24, 32–33.

Nelkin, Dorothy, and Michael S. Brown. 1984. *Workers at Risk: Voices from the Workplace.* Chicago: University of Chicago Press.

Nietzsche, Friedrich. 1987. *The Gay Science.* New York: Vintage Books.

Parks, David. 1993a. "Gulf Vets Complain VA Too Slow with Benefits." *Birmingham News,* March 19.

———. 1993b. "Survey of Gulf Vets' Ills Surprises VA." *Birmingham News,* September 19.

———. 1996a. "Gulf War Nightmare Lives on for Veteran." *Birmingham News,* July 8.

———. 1996b. "Key Senators Clash Over Gulf Illnesses." *Birmingham News,* July 17.

Parsons, Talcott. 1951. *The Social System.* Glencoe, IL: Free Press.

Pullman, Cydney, and Sharon Szymanski. 1993. *Multiple Chemical Sensitivities at Work: A Training Workbook for Working People.* New York: The Labor Institute of New York.

Rest, Kathleen M. 1995. "A Survey of AOEC Physician Practices and Attitudes Regarding Multiple Chemical Sensitivity." In *Multiple Chemical*

Sensitivity: A Scientific Overview, edited by Frank L. Mitchell, 51–66. Washington, DC: U.S. Department of Health and Human Services and ATSDR.

Sagan, Carl. 1996. *The Demon-Haunted World: Science as a Candle in the Dark.* New York: Random House.

Samet, Jonathan, and Devra Lee Davis. 1995. "Introduction." In *Multiple Chemical Sensitivity: A Scientific Overview,* edited by Frank L. Mitchell, 1–3. U.S. Department of Health and Human Services. Princeton, NJ: Princeton Scientific Publishing.

Schnaiberg, Alan. 1980. *The Environment: From Surplus to Scarcity.* New York: Oxford University Press.

Schutz, Alfred. 1967. *The Phenomenology of the Social World.* Chicago: Northwestern University Press.

Seligman, Adam B. 1992. *The Ideal of Civil Society.* Princeton, NJ: Princeton University Press.

Selner, John. 1988. "Chemical Sensitivity." In *Current Therapy in Allergy, Immunology, and Rheumatology,* edited by Lawrence M. Lichtenstein and Anthony S. Fauci, 48–52. Toronto: B. C. Decker.

———. 1991. "Editorial." *Chemecology* 20:1–3.

Sheets-Johnstone, Maxine, ed. 1992. *Giving the Body Its Due.* Albany: State University of New York Press.

Simon, Gregory E. 1995. "Epidemic Multiple Chemical Sensitivity after an Outbreak of Sick-Building Syndrome." In *Multiple Chemical Sensitivity: A Scientific Overview,* edited by Frank L. Mitchell, 41–46. Washington, DC: U.S. Department of Health and Human Services and ATSDR.

Simon, Gregory E., Wayne J. Katon, and Patricia J. Sparks. 1990. "Allergic to Life: Psychological Factors in Environmental Illness." *American Journal of Psychiatry,* 147:901–6.

Sontag, Susan. 1989. *Illness as Metaphor.* New York: Anchor.

Stanley, J. S. 1986. "Broad Scan Analysis of Human Adipose Tissue, Executive Summary, Vol. 1." EPA Contract—560/5-86/035. Springfield, VA: National Technical Information Service.

Starr, Paul. 1982. *The Social Transformation of American Medicine.* New York: Basic Books.

Stewart, Charles, Craig Smith, and Robert Denton Jr. 1984. *Persuasion and Social Movements.* Prospects Heights, IL: Waveland Press.

Szasz, Andrew. 1994. *EcoPopulism.* Minneapolis: University of Minnesota Press.

Terr, Abba J. 1987. "Multiple Chemical Sensitivities: Immunological Critique of Clinical Ecology Theories and Practice." *Occupational Medicine: State of the Art Reviews* 2:683–94.

Thomas, Keith. 1983. *Man and the Natural World.* London: Allen Lane.

Touraine, Alain. 1995. *Critique of Modernity.* Oxford: Blackwell.

Turner, Bryan S. 1984. *The Body and Society.* Oxford: Blackwell.

———. 1995. *Medical Power and Social Knowledge.* London: Sage.

United Methodist Church, General Board of Global Ministries. 1994. *United Methodist Resource Book about Accessibility.* New York: United Methodist Church.

U.S. Department of Energy. 1991. Public Hearing, Report No. 503-23-564. Washington, DC.

U.S. Department of Labor. 1988. OSHA 3111-Hazard Communication Guidelines for Compliance, 1–13. Washington, DC: OSHA.

U.S. Environmental Protection Agency. 1980. Hazardous Waste Facility Siting: A Critical Problem (SW-865). Washington, DC: U.S. Government Printing Office.

U.S. House of Representatives Subcommittee on Oversight and Investigations, 1993.

U.S. Senate Subcommittee. 1989. Indoor Air Quality Act, 3 May 1989 (S. Hrg. 101-2). Washington, DC: U.S. Government Printing Office.

Waltzer, Michael. 1991. "The Idea of Civil Society." *Dissent,* spring, 293–304.

West, Jane. 1993. "The Evolution of Disability Rights." In *Implementing the Americans with Disabilities Act: Rights and Responsibilities of All Americans,* edited by Lawrence O. Gostin and Henry A. Beyer, 3–15. Baltimore: Paul H. Brooks.

Wilson, Cynthia. 1995. "Clueless in Bethesda." *Our Toxic Times* 6, no. 6:1–4.

World Almanac. 1997. Mahwah, NJ: K-III Reference Corporation.

Wright, Will. 1992. *Wild Knowledge.* Minneapolis: University of Minnesota Press.

Young, Allen. 1971. "Internalizing and Externalizing Medical Belief Systems: An Ethiopian Example." *Social Science Medicine* 10:147–56.

———. 1976. "Some Implications of Medical Beliefs and Practices for Social Anthropology." *American Anthropologist* 78:5–24.

———. 1982. "The Anthropologies of Illness and Sickness." *Annual Review of Anthropology* 11:257–85.

Name Index

Atkinson, Paul, 55

Baudrillard, Jean, 172
Bauman, Zygmunt, 10, 61
Beck, Ulrich, 5, 5–6, 7–8, 9, 10, 57, 87,
    91–92, 111–112, 117–118, 150, 201,
    202
Berger, Peter, 9, 47, 72
Berger and Luckman, 9, 47, 72
Bickerton, Derek, 89
Brown, Michael S., 8, 170
Brown, Phil, 192, 194
Burke, Kenneth, 49, 92, 111

Calhoun, Craig, 40
Carson, Rachel, 3
Conrad, Peter, 61–62
Conrad and Schneider, 61–62
Couch, Stephen R., 9, 149
Couch and Kroll-Smith, 9, 149
Crumpler, Diana, 3, 41

Denton, Robert, Jr., 136
Denzin, Norman, 82
DiGacomo, Susan, 4
Dossey, Larry, 60, 118
Douglas, Mary, 73, 178, 202
Dubos, Rene, 1–2
Dumont, Louis, 61
Dunlap, Riley E., 186–187
Dunlap, Gallup, and Gallup, 186–187
Durkheim, Emile, 73, 145, 150, 178

Engle, George L., 60, 117
Epstein, Steven, 8, 135

Figlio, Karl, 143
Foucault, Michel, 6, 18, 32, 37, 93, 104,
    131, 132, 187, 190
Frank, Arthur, 198, 199–200, 205, 207
Freund, Peter E. S., 1–2, 21 37, 60,
    104–105, 170, 192
Freund and McGuire, 1–2, 21, 37, 60,
    104–105, 170, 192

Gallup, Alec M., 186–187
Gallup, George H., Jr., 186–187
Geertz, Clifford, 11, 38, 50, 110, 131,
    145, 180
Gibbs, Lois Marie, 190–191, 193, 195
Giddens, Anthony, 5, 5–6, 8, 57, 58, 72,
    87, 107, 136, 147, 151
Gordon, Deborah R., 60
Gusfield, Joseph, 135, 136

Habermas, Jurgen, 59
Harvey, David, 32

Irwin, Alan, 191, 194, 198–199, 207

Johnstone, Albert A., 60

Kafka, Franz, 87, 206
Kosak, David, 134
Kroll-Smith, Steve, 9, 21, 21–22, 72,
    149, 205
Kroll-Smith and Ladd, 21, 21–22, 149,
    205
Kuhn, Thomas, 96, 198, 200, 201, 202

Ladd, Anthony, 21, 21–22, 205

Subject Index